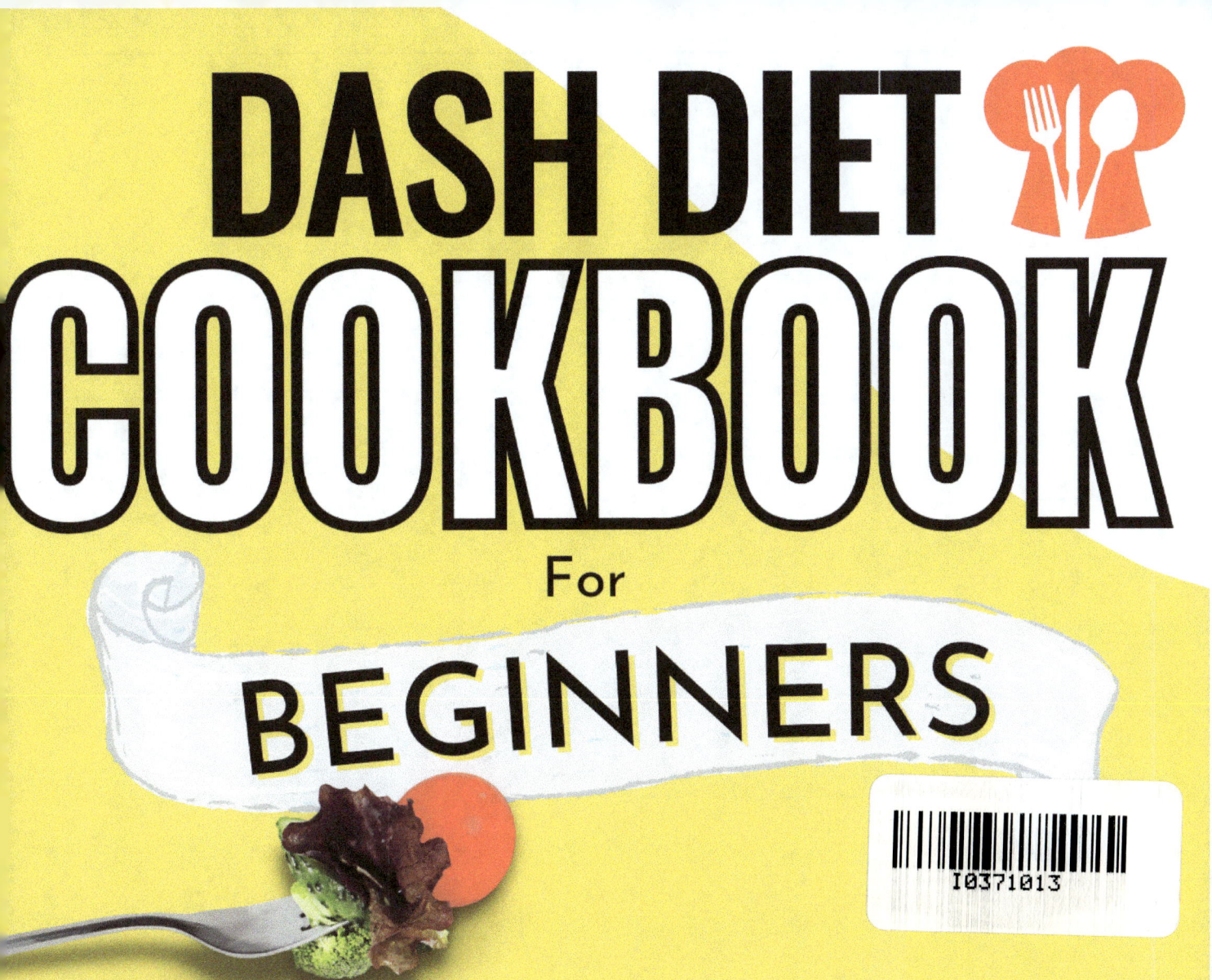

DASH DIET COOKBOOK For BEGINNERS

LOW-FAT RECIPES TO PROMOTE WEIGHT LOSS, LOWER BLOOD PRESSURE, AND HELP PREVENT DIABETES

-VANESSA TINGEY-

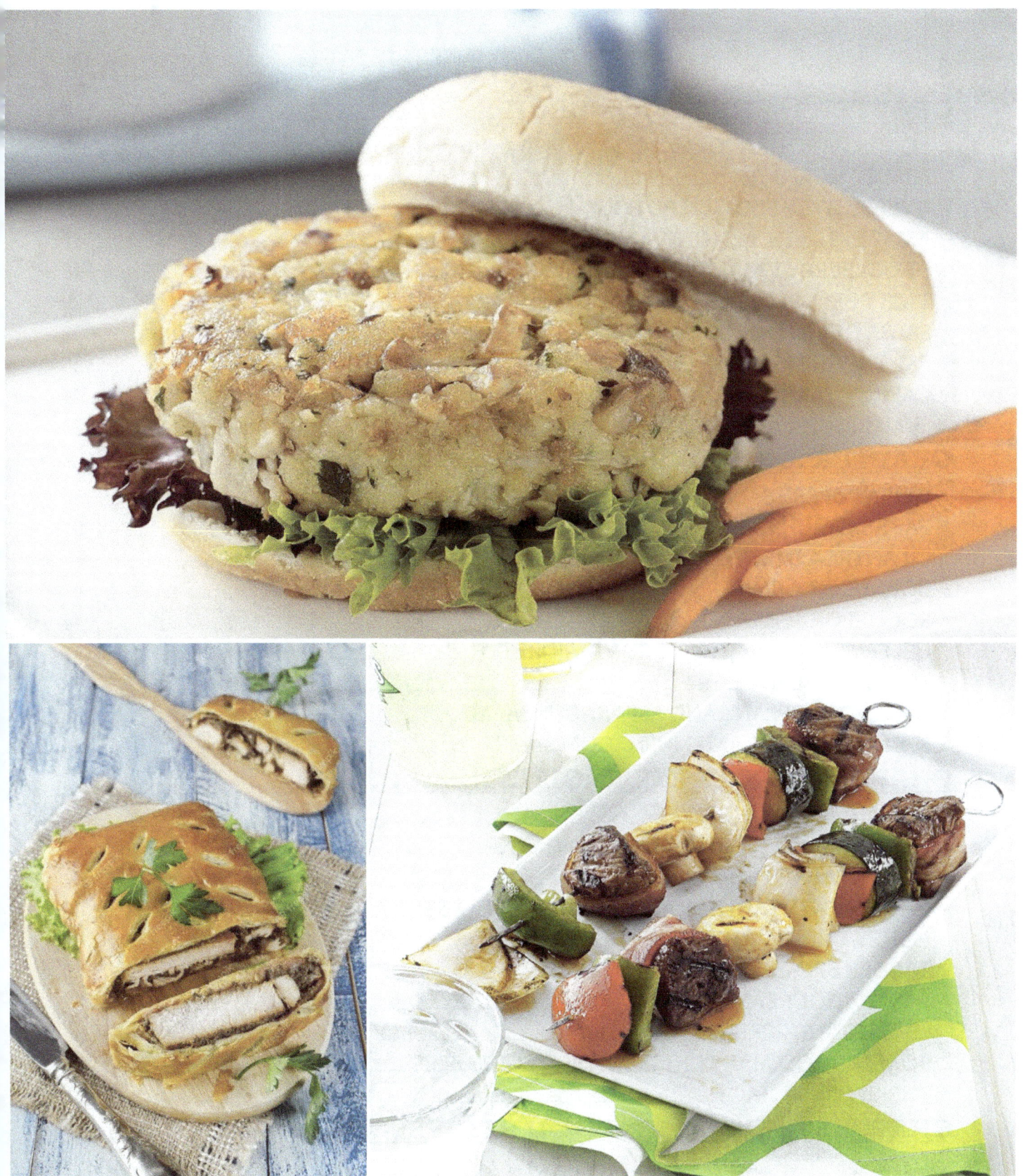

TABLE OF CONTENTS:

CHAPTER 1: BREAKFAST RECIPES 8
- YOGURT AND GRANOLA 9
- MILLET MUFFINS 11
- CHEESY OVEN SCRAMBLED EGGS 13
- AMAZING DATE, ALMOND, AND YOGURT BREAD 15
- STRAWBERRY VANILLA PANCAKES 18
- TASTY BELL PEPPER FRITTATA 20
- SALSA DEVILED EGGS 23
- FANTASTIC MORNING GLORY MUFFINS 25
- CARROT CAKE QUINOA 28
- SUMMER CHICKPEA SALAD 30

CHAPTER 2: SALAD RECIPES 33
- WHEAT BERRY SALAD 34
- FAST SRIRACHA TUNA SALAD 36
- CILANTRO-LIME STEAK SALAD 38
- CORNUCOPIA SALAD 41
- ROQUEFORT PEAR SALAD 44
- CELERY SALAD WITH SHERRY VINAIGRETTE 47
- TSIMMES SALAD 49
- GRILLED EGGPLANT AND ASPARAGUS SALAD 50
- SPINACH, BACON, AND MUSHROOM SALAD 53

CHAPTER 3: POULTRY RECIPES 56
- SPICY HOT CHICKEN LEGS 57
- CHICKEN NAPA CABBAGE WRAPS 59
- TURKEY WRAPS 61
- CHICKEN WITH ARTICHOKES AND GOAT CHEESE 64
- HONEY-GARLIC CHICKEN THIGHS 67
- TENDER BREADED TURKEY CUTLETS 70
- FANTASTIC CREAMY ALMOND CHICKEN BAKE 72
- FIVE SPICE CHICKEN 75
- ROASTED ROSEMARY CHICKEN AND VEGETABLES 78
- TURKEY CHILI MAC 81

CHAPTER 4: FISH & SEAFOOD RECIPES 86

AMAZING TUNA BURGERS 87
SALMON WITH DILL 89
GARLICKY SHRIMP SCAMPI 91
GRILLED PESTO SHRIMP SKEWERS 93
STUFFED SOLE WITH IMITATION CRAB 95

CHAPTER 5: SOUP & STEW RECIPES 99
ASPARAGUS SOUP 100
CHICKPEA SOUP 102
SEAFOOD STEW 104
VEGAN CREAM OF ASPARAGUS SOUP 106
GREEN DETOX SOUP 109

CHAPTER 6: MEAT RECIPES 113
BEEF PEPPER STEAK 114
PORK TENDERLOIN WITH TOMATO AND PEPPER SAUCE 116
AMAZING RICE AND BEEF STUFFED TOMATOES 119
KOREAN BEEF WITH CAULI RICE 122
VEGGIE AND BEEF CHILI 124

CHAPTER 7: VEGETABLE AND GRAIN RECIPES 128
VEGGIE PITA PIZZA 129
CURRY TOFU STIR-FRY 131
LENTILS AND SPINACH 133
LIMA BEAN HUMMUS 136
VEGAN CHILI VERDE 138

© Copyright 2021 by Vanessa Tingey All rights reserved.

The following Book is reproduced below with the goal of providing information that is as accurate and reliable as possible. Regardless, purchasing this Book can be seen as consent to the fact that both the publisher and the author of this book are in no way experts on the topics discussed within and that any recommendations or suggestions that are made herein are for entertainment purposes only. Professionals should be consulted as needed prior to undertaking any of the action endorsed herein.

This declaration is deemed fair and valid by both the American Bar Association and the Committee of Publishers Association and is legally binding throughout the United States.

Furthermore, the transmission, duplication, or reproduction of any of the following work including specific information will be considered an illegal act irrespective of if it is done electronically or in print. This extends to creating a secondary or tertiary copy of the work or a recorded copy and is only allowed with the express written consent from the Publisher. All additional right reserved.

The information in the following pages is broadly considered a truthful and accurate account of facts and as such, any inattention, use, or misuse of the information in question by the reader will render any resulting actions solely under their purview. There are no scenarios in which the publisher or the original author of this work can be in any fashion deemed liable for any hardship or damages that may befall them after undertaking information described herein.

Additionally, the information in the following pages is intended only for informational purposes and should thus be thought of as universal. As befitting its nature, it is presented without assurance regarding its prolonged validity or interim quality. Trademarks that are mentioned are done without written consent and can in no way be considered

an endorsement from the trademark holder.

CHAPTER 1: BREAKFAST RECIPES

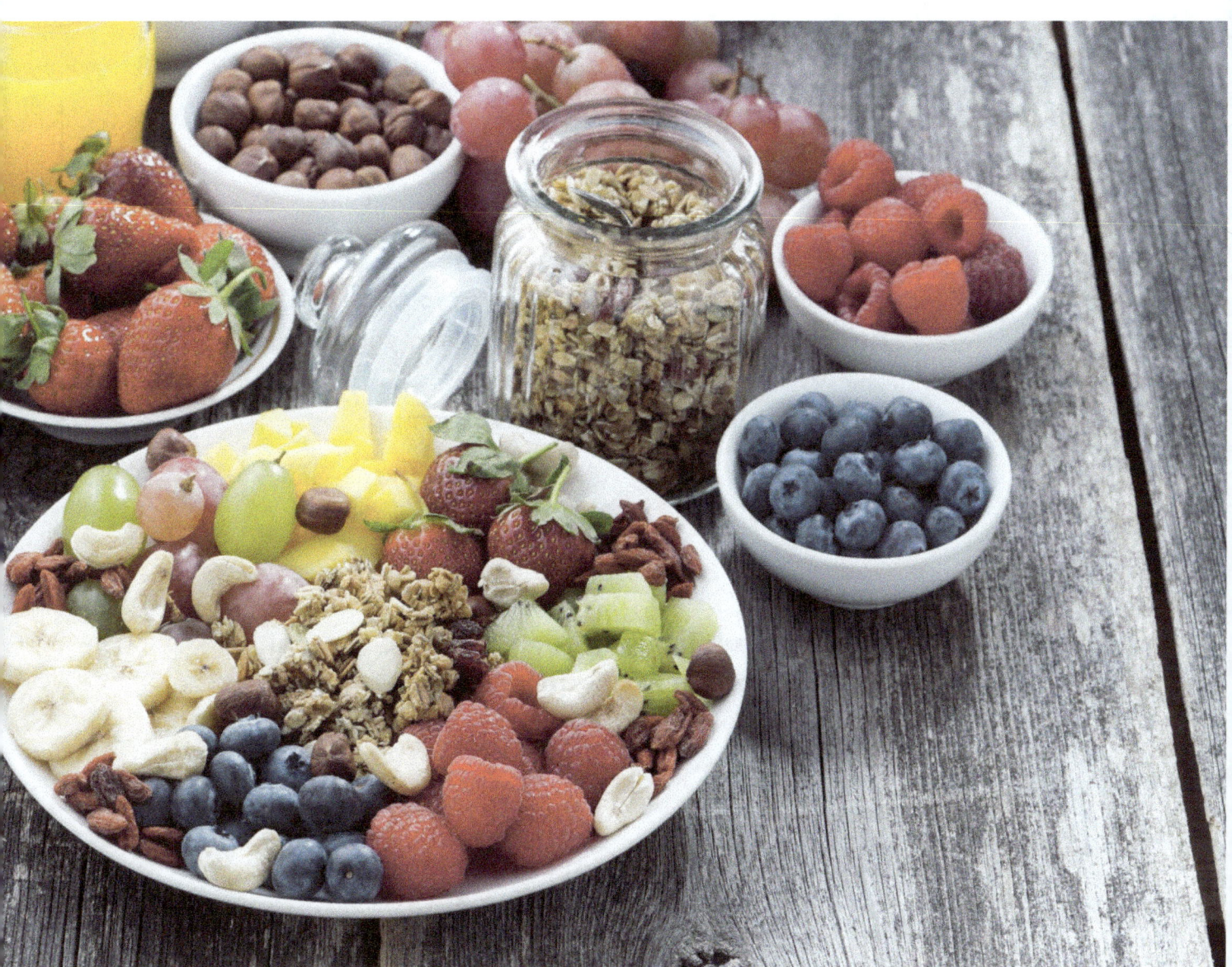

YOGURT AND GRANOLA

Prep:
5 mins
Total:
5 mins
Servings:
1
Yield:
1 serving

INGREDIENTS:

1 tablespoon flaxseed meal
1 pinch ground cinnamon, or to taste
1 (6 ounce) container fat-free plain yogurt
¼ cup granola
1 tablespoon light agave syrup

DIRECTIONS:

1
Stir yogurt, granola, agave syrup, flaxseed meal, and cinnamon together in a bowl.

NUTRITION FACTS:

344 calories; protein 15.6g; carbohydrates 48.1g; fat 10.6g; cholesterol 3.4mg;

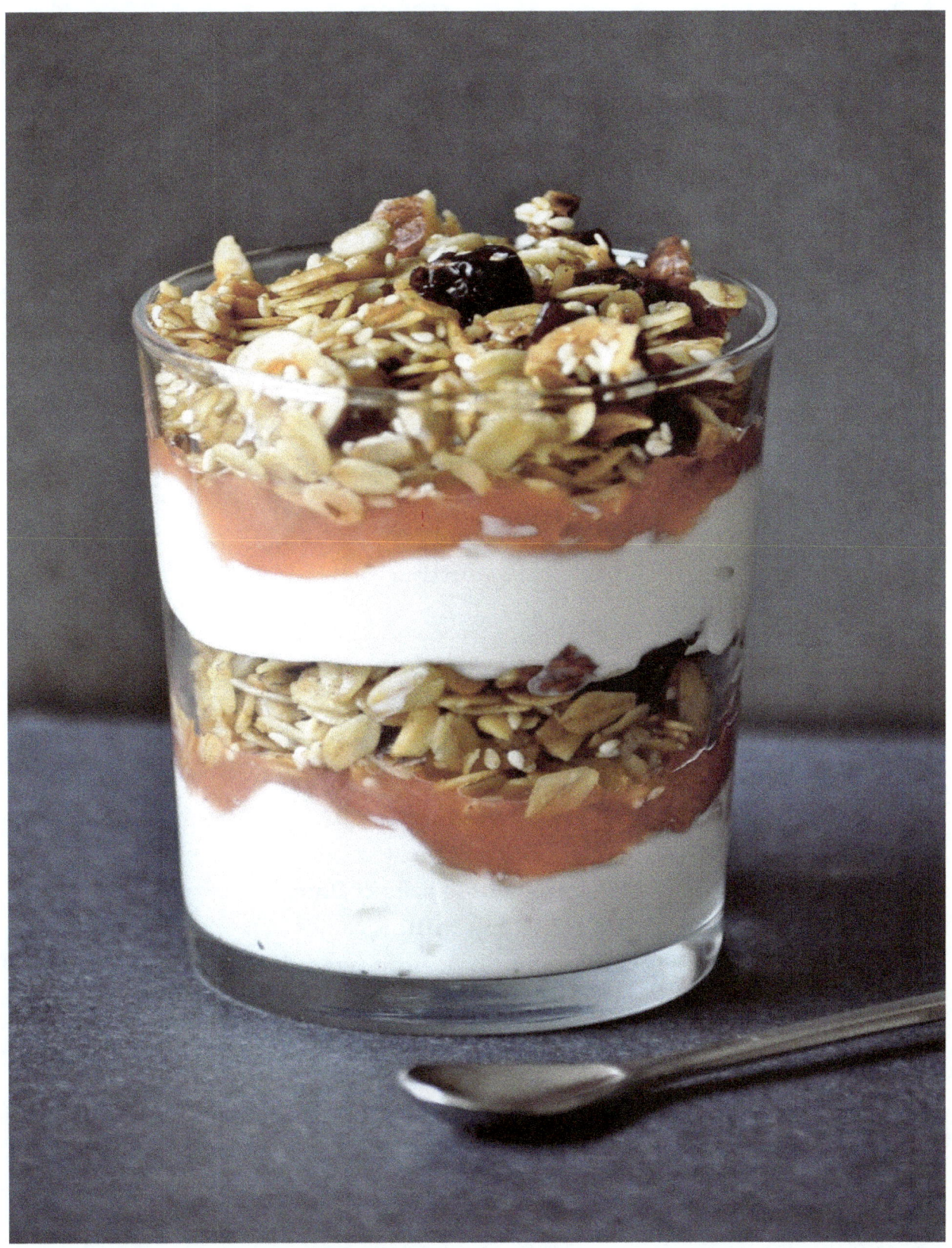

MILLET MUFFINS

Prep:
10 mins
Cook:
15 mins
Total:
25 mins
Servings:
16
Yield:
16 muffins

INGREDIENTS:

1 cup buttermilk
1 egg, lightly beaten
½ cup vegetable oil
½ cup honey
2 ¼ cups whole wheat flour
⅓ cup millet
1 teaspoon baking powder
1 teaspoon baking soda
1 teaspoon salt

DIRECTIONS:

1

Preheat oven to 400 degrees F (200 degrees C).
Grease 16 muffin cups.

2

In a large bowl, mix the whole wheat flour,
millet flour, baking powder, baking soda, and salt.
In a separate bowl, mix the buttermilk,
egg, vegetable oil, and honey.
Stir buttermilk mixture into the flour mixture
just until evenly moist.
Transfer batter to the prepared muffin cups.

3

Bake 15 minutes in the preheated oven,
or until a toothpick inserted
in the center of a muffin comes out clean

NUTRITION FACTS:

176 calories; protein 3.7g; carbohydrates 24.8g; fat 7.7g; cholesterol 12.2mg;

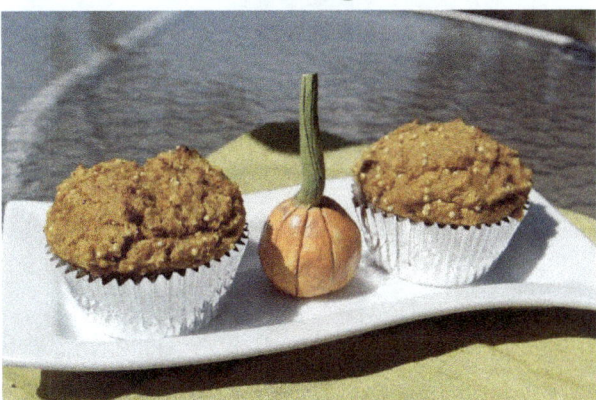

CHEESY OVEN SCRAMBLED EGGS

Prep:
10 mins
Cook:
30 mins
Total:
40 mins
Servings:
18
Yield:
1 13x9-inch dish

INGREDIENTS:

⅓ cup butter, melted
24 eggs
2 ¼ teaspoons seasoned salt
2 teaspoons hot pepper sauce
2 teaspoons mustard powder
2 cups milk
1 ½ cups shredded sharp Cheddar cheese

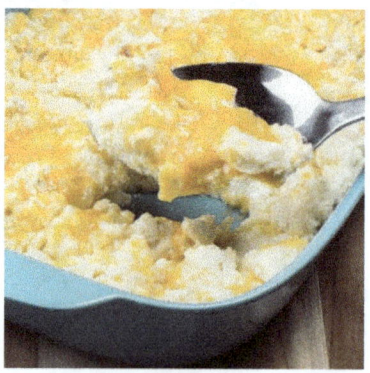

DIRECTIONS:

1

Preheat oven to 350 degrees F (175 degrees C).

2

Pour melted butter into a glass 9x13-inch baking dish.
Tilt dish to coat bottom with butter.

3

Beat eggs, Cheddar cheese, seasoned salt, hot pepper sauce,
and mustard powder together with a whisk in a large bowl.
Stream milk into egg mixture while whisking;
pour into the baking dish.

4

Bake in preheated oven for 15 minutes, stir,
and continue baking until eggs are set in the middle,
15 to 20 minutes more. Serve immediately.

NUTRITION FACTS:

188 calories; protein 12.3g; carbohydrates 2.1g; fat 14.5g;

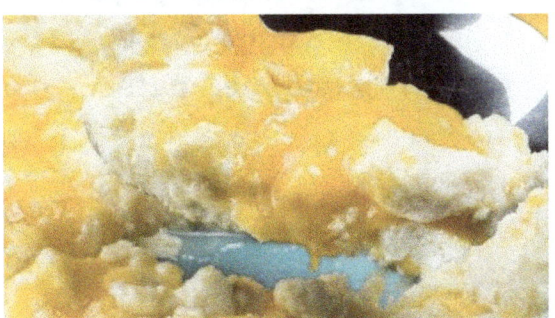

AMAZING DATE, ALMOND, AND YOGURT BREAD

Prep:
15 mins
Cook:
55 mins
Total:
1 hr 10 mins
Servings:
8
Yield:
1 6-inch cake

INGREDIENTS:

¾ cup slivered almonds
1 cup white sugar
2 cups all-purpose flour
1 teaspoon baking soda
1 teaspoon ground nutmeg
½ teaspoon salt
½ cup butter, softened
¾ cup whole milk yogurt
2 eggs
1 cup chopped dates

DIRECTIONS:

1

Preheat oven to 350 degrees F (175 degrees C). Grease a 6-inch baking pan.

2

Spread almonds on a baking sheet.

3

Toast almonds in the preheated oven until they turn golden brown and become fragrant, about 5 minutes.

4

Combine sugar and butter in a large bowl; beat with an electric mixer until creamy. Beat in yogurt and eggs.
Mix in flour, baking soda, nutmeg, and salt.
Fold 1/2 cup toasted almonds and dates into the batter.

5

Pour batter into the prepared pan. Top with remaining 1/4 cup toasted almonds.

6

Bake in the preheated oven until a toothpick inserted into the center comes out clean, 50 to 60 minutes.

NUTRITION FACTS:

470 calories; protein 8.4g; carbohydrates 68.9g; fat 19.2g;

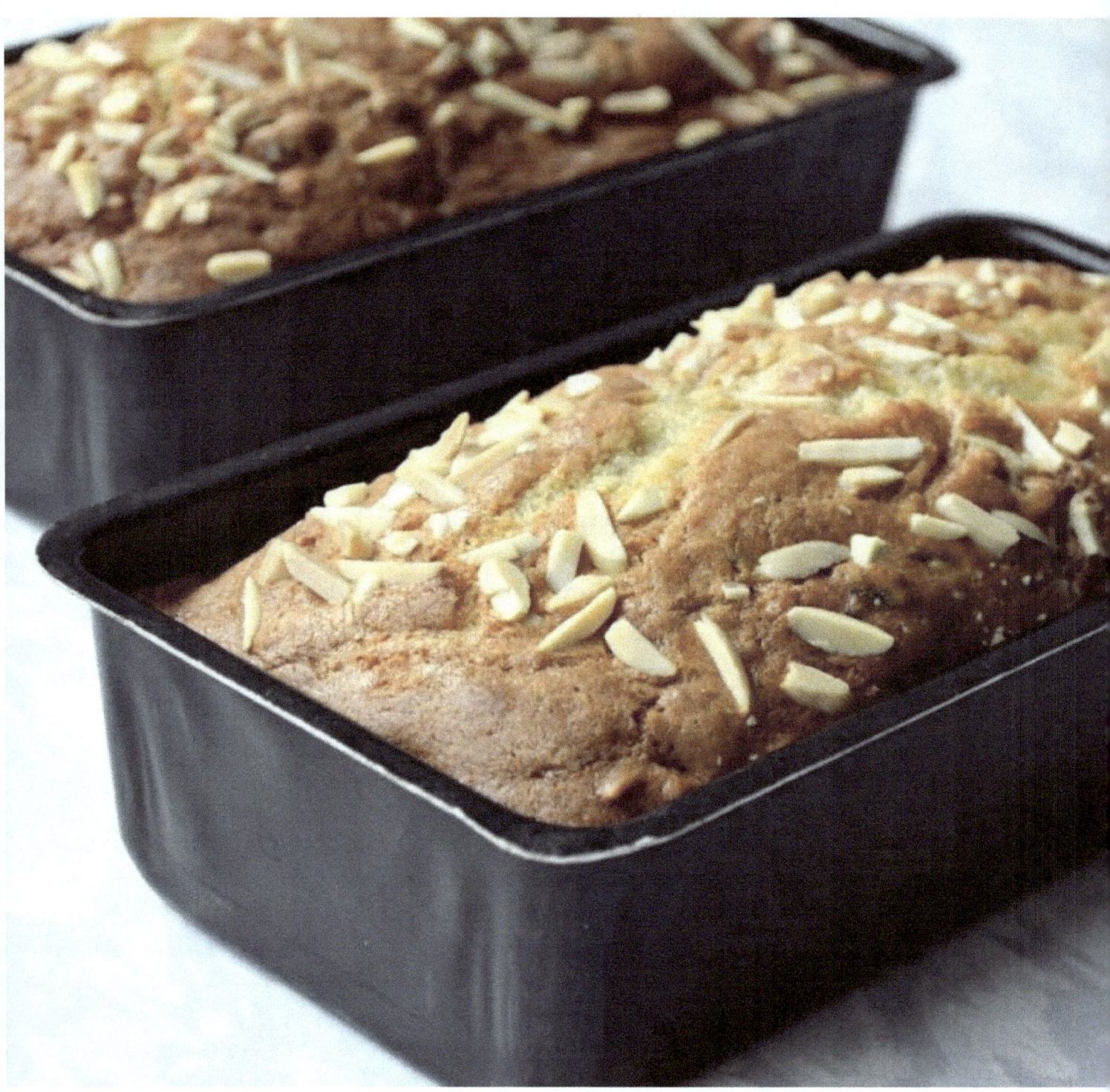

STRAWBERRY VANILLA PANCAKES

Prep:
10 mins
Cook:
10 mins
Total:
20 mins
Servings:
4
Yield:
8 pancakes

INGREDIENTS:

1 cup milk
2 tablespoons vegetable oil
2 tablespoons vanilla extract
1 cup chopped fresh strawberries
1 cup all-purpose flour
2 tablespoons brown sugar
2 teaspoons baking powder
1 teaspoon salt
1 egg

DIRECTIONS:

1

In a medium bowl, stir together the flour,
brown sugar,
baking powder and salt. Pour in the milk,
oil, egg and vanilla, and mix until well blended.
Stir in the strawberries.

2

Heat a large skillet
or griddle over medium heat,
and coat with butter or cooking spray.
Pour batter into desired size of pancakes.
Flip with a spatula when bubbles
appear in the center.
Cook until golden brown on the other side.

NUTRITION FACTS:

280 calories; protein 7.1g; carbohydrates 37.7g;
fat 9.7g; cholesterol 51.4mg;

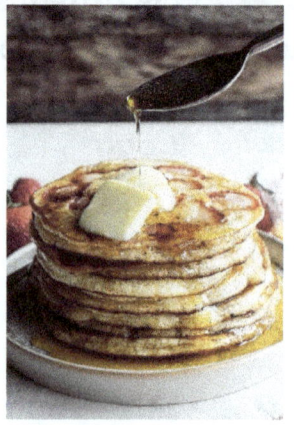

TASTY BELL PEPPER FRITTATA

Prep:
15 mins
Cook:
1 hr 5 mins
Total:
1 hr 20 mins
Servings:
1
Yield:
1 serving

INGREDIENTS:

1 pinch dried basil, or to taste
1 pinch salt and ground black pepper to taste
1 teaspoon shredded Cheddar cheese, or to taste
1 large red bell pepper, top and seeds removed
1 teaspoon butter (Optional)
1 tablespoon chopped onion
1 roma (plum) tomato, seeded and chopped
2 eggs, beaten
1 teaspoon butter (Optional)
1 pinch dried tarragon, or to taste

DIRECTIONS:

1

Preheat oven to 350 degrees F (175 degrees C).

2

Heat the butter in a skillet over medium heat until the foam subsides, and cook and stir the onion and tomato until the onion is translucent and the liquid from the tomato has evaporated, about 8 minutes. Transfer the tomato and onion to a bowl. Pour the beaten eggs into the cooked vegetables, and stir in tarragon, basil, salt, black pepper, and Cheddar cheese until thoroughly combined. Pour the egg mixture into the red bell pepper, and set into a small baking dish, standing upright. Cover the dish and pepper with foil.

3

Bake in the preheated oven until the pepper is tender and the eggs are set, about 55 minutes.

NUTRITION FACTS:

307 calories; protein 16.6g; carbohydrates 15.1g; fat 20.4g;

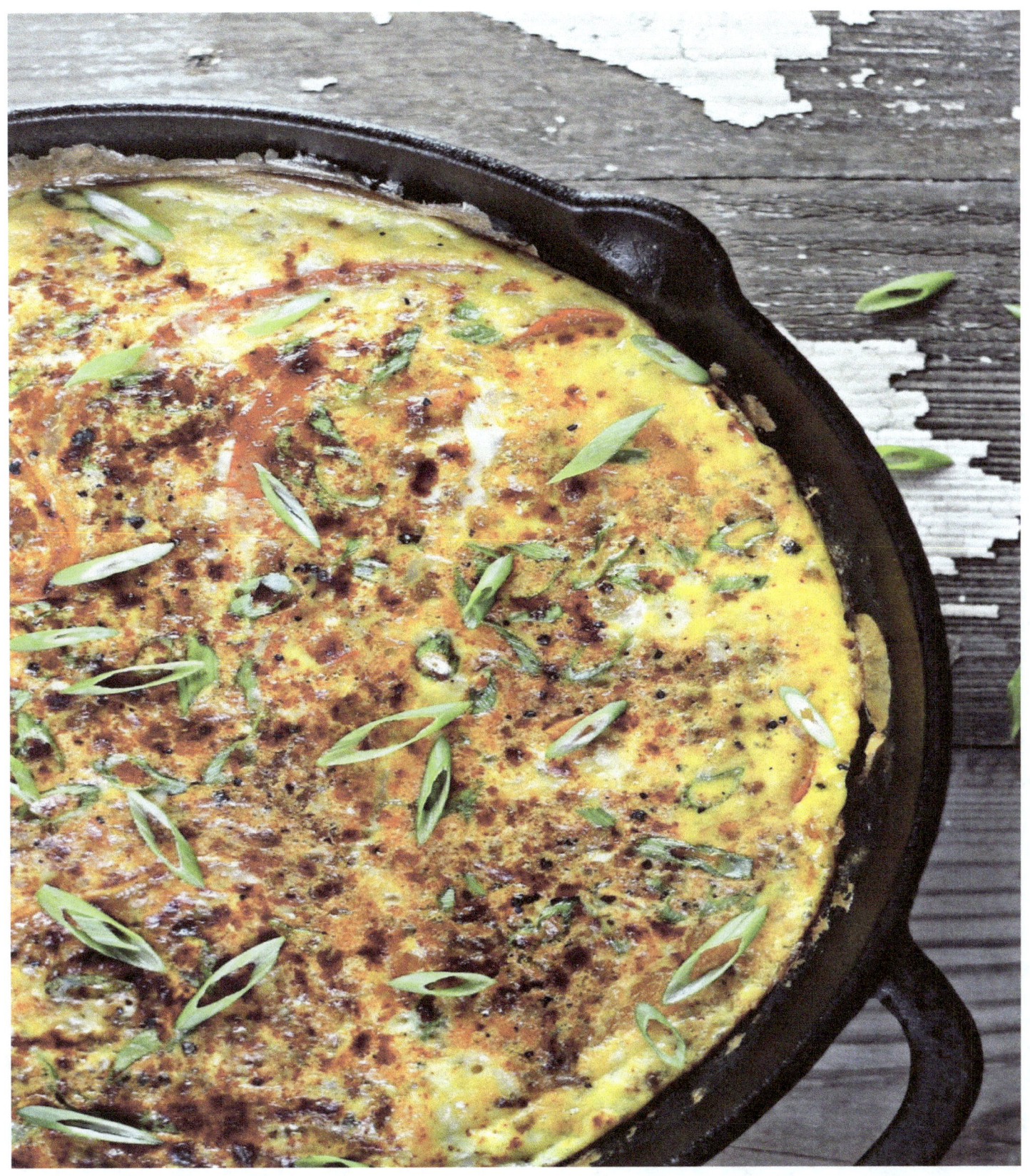

SALSA DEVILED EGGS

Prep:
30 mins
Total:
30 mins
Servings:
12
Yield:
12 servings

INGREDIENTS:

Eggs:

6 Eggland's Best Eggs, hard cooked and peeled
3 tablespoons fresh salsa or chunky salsa, drained, if necessary
1 tablespoon sour cream

Topping:

2 teaspoons fresh salsa
1 teaspoon Chopped fresh cilantro

DIRECTIONS:

1

Cut eggs in half lengthwise. Remove egg yolks; place yolks into bowl.

2

Mash yolks with fork. Add 3 tablespoons salsa and sour cream; mix well.

3

Spoon about 1 tablespoon egg yolk mixture into each egg white half.

4

Top each with about 1/2 teaspoon salsa and garnish with cilantro, if desired.

5

Cover and refrigerate until serving time or up to 24 hours.

NUTRITION FACTS:

35 calories; protein 2.9g; carbohydrates 0.5g; fat 2.4g; cholesterol 93.6mg; sodium 61.1mg.

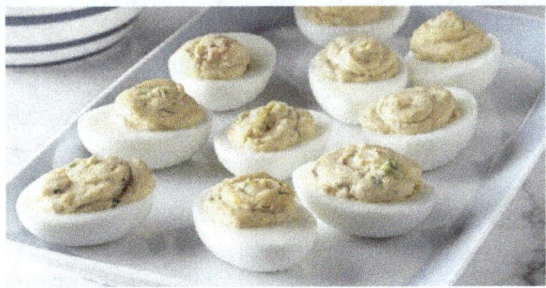

FANTASTIC MORNING GLORY MUFFINS

Prep:
15 mins
Cook:
20 mins
Total:
35 mins
Servings:
18
Yield:
18 muffins

INGREDIENTS:

1 ½ cups all-purpose flour
½ cup whole wheat flour
1 ¼ cups white sugar
1 tablespoon ground cinnamon
2 teaspoons baking powder
½ teaspoon baking soda
½ teaspoon salt
2 cups grated carrots
1 apple - peeled, cored, and chopped
1 cup raisins
1 egg

2 egg whites
½ cup apple butter
¼ cup vegetable oil
1 tablespoon vanilla extract
2 tablespoons chopped walnuts
2 tablespoons toasted wheat germ

DIRECTIONS:

1
Preheat oven to 375 degrees F (190 degrees C).
Lightly oil 18 muffin cups,
or coat with nonstick cooking spray.

2
In a medium bowl, whisk together eggs,
egg whites, apple butter, oil and vanilla.

3
In a large bowl, stir together flours,
sugar, cinnamon,
baking powder,
baking soda and salt.
Stir in carrots,
apples and raisins.
Stir in apple butter
mixture until just moistened. Spoon the batter
into the prepared muffin cups,
filling them about 3/4 full.

4

In a small bowl, combine walnuts and wheat germ; sprinkle over the muffin tops.

5

Bake at 375 degrees F (190 degrees C) for 15 to 20 minutes, or until the tops are golden and spring back when lightly pressed.

NUTRITION FACTS:

194 calories; protein 3.1g; carbohydrates 37.3g; fat 4.2g; cholesterol 10.3mg;

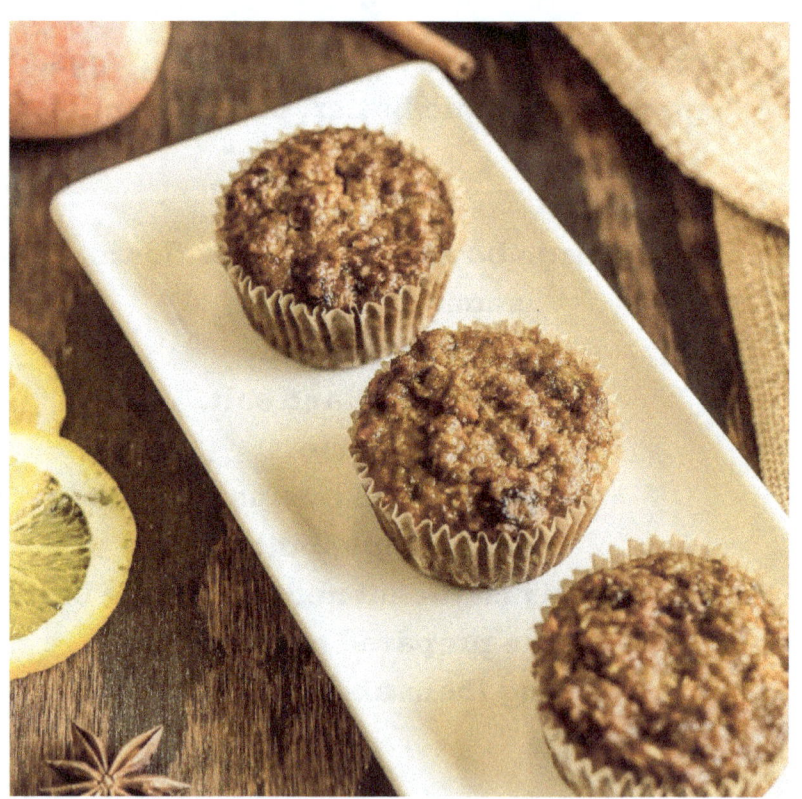

CARROT CAKE QUINOA

Prep:
10 mins
Cook:
20 mins
Additional:
5 mins
Total:
35 mins
Servings:
4
Yield:
4 servings

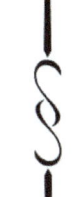

INGREDIENTS:

4 cups water
1 cup quinoa
¾ cup amaranth
¼ cup wild rice
2 teaspoons ground cumin
1 teaspoon salt
2 stalks celery, diced
1 large carrot, grated
½ cup canned chickpeas (garbanzo beans) (Optional)
½ cup raisins
1 tablespoon olive oil
1 clove garlic, minced
salt and ground black pepper to taste

DIRECTIONS:

1
Bring water, quinoa, amaranth, wild rice, cumin, and 1 teaspoon salt to a boil in a saucepan. Reduce heat to medium-low, cover, and simmer until grains are tender and water has been absorbed, 20 to 25 minutes. Let stand for 5 minutes.

2
Mix celery, carrot, chickpeas, raisins, olive oil, garlic, salt, and pepper together in a bowl; add grain mixture and mix well.

NUTRITION FACTS:

472 calories; protein 15.4g; carbohydrates 85.1g; fat 9.2g;

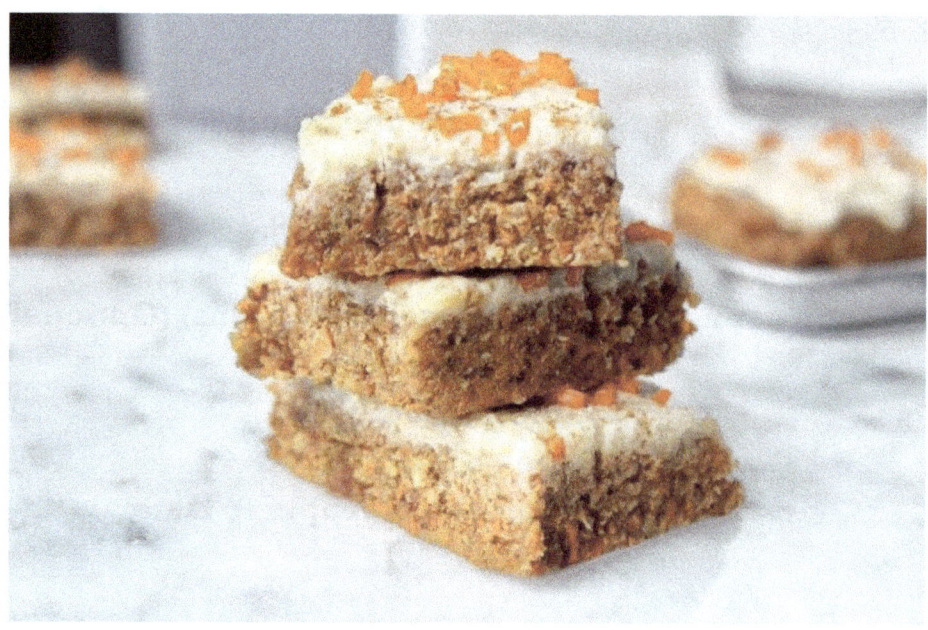

SUMMER CHICKPEA SALAD

Prep:
15 mins
Cook:
1 min
Additional:
1 hr
Total:
1 hr 16 mins
Servings:
6
Yield:
6 servings

INGREDIENTS:

2 (19 ounce) cans chickpeas (garbanzos), drained and rinsed
1 pint small cherry tomatoes, halved
3 tablespoons finely shredded basil leaves
½ cup crumbled goat-milk feta cheese
2 tablespoons honey
3 large cloves garlic, minced
3 tablespoons red wine vinegar
3 tablespoons cider vinegar
3 tablespoons olive oil
½ teaspoon ground black pepper
¼ teaspoon cayenne pepper
¼ teaspoon salt

DIRECTIONS:

1
Toss chickpeas, tomatoes, feta cheese,
and basil together in a large mixing bowl.

2
Put honey in a small glass bowl;
heat in microwave 30 seconds.
Stir garlic, red wine vinegar, cider vinegar, olive oil,
black pepper, cayenne pepper,
and salt with the honey to make a dressing;
pour over the chickpea
salad and toss to coat.

3
Cover the mixing bowl with plastic wrap.
Refrigerate salad for 1 hour before serving.

NUTRITION FACTS:

347 calories; protein 11.4g; carbohydrates 50.9g; fat 11.7g;

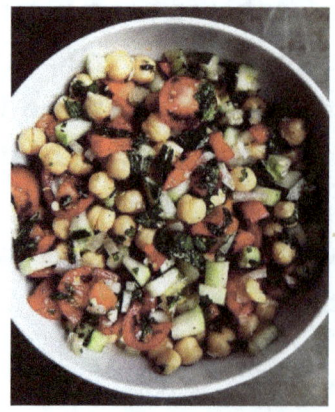

CHAPTER 2: SALAD RECIPES

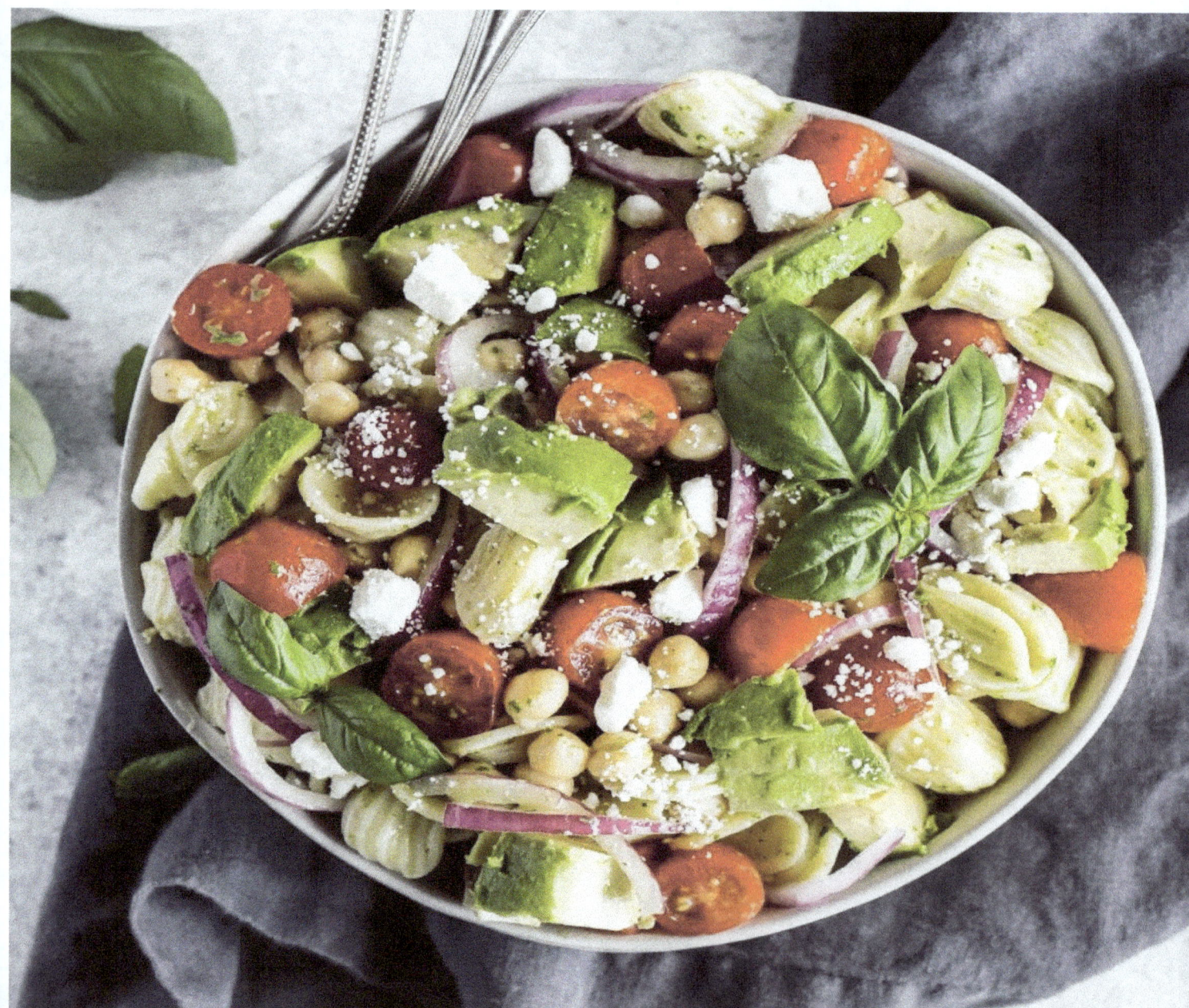

WHEAT BERRY SALAD

Prep:
15 mins
Cook:
1 hr
Additional:
3 hrs 20 mins
Total:
4 hrs 35 mins
Servings:
6
Yield:
6 servings

INGREDIENTS:

1 cup wheat berries
4 cups water
2 carrots, diced
1 stalk celery, diced
¼ white onion, diced
¼ cup chopped fresh parsley
2 tablespoons lemon juice
1 tablespoon soy sauce
1 tablespoon tahini
1 tablespoon olive oil
1 tablespoon honey, or more to taste
salt to taste

DIRECTIONS:

1
Place wheat berries in a pot and cover with water;
soak for 3 to 6 hours.

2
Drain wheat berries and add 4 cups water;
bring to a boil.
Reduce heat and simmer until wheat berries
are tender yet firm
to the bite and water is absorbed, 1 to 2 hours.
Remove pot from heat and cool.

3
Mix carrots, celery, onion, and parsley into wheat berries.

4
Whisk lemon juice, soy sauce, tahini, olive oil,
honey, and salt together in a bowl until smooth;
stir into wheat berries mixture.

NUTRITION FACTS:

167 calories; protein 5.1g; carbohydrates 30g; fat 4.2g;

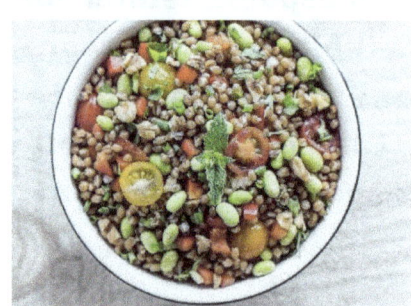

FAST SRIRACHA TUNA SALAD

Prep:
10 mins
Additional:
5 mins
Total:
15 mins
Servings:
2
Yield:
2 servings

INGREDIENTS:

3 mini sweet peppers, or more to taste
2 tablespoons Sriracha hot chili sauce, or more to taste
2 tablespoons mayonnaise
1 (5 ounce) can tuna, or more to taste, drained and flaked
2 hard-boiled eggs, chopped
2 tablespoons honey mustard

DIRECTIONS:

1

Mix tuna, eggs, and peppers in a bowl. Stir sriracha, mayonnaise, and honey mustard into the tuna mixture.

2

Refrigerate tuna salad for 5 minutes.

NUTRITION FACTS:

303 calories; protein 23.6g; carbohydrates 12g; fat 17.9g;

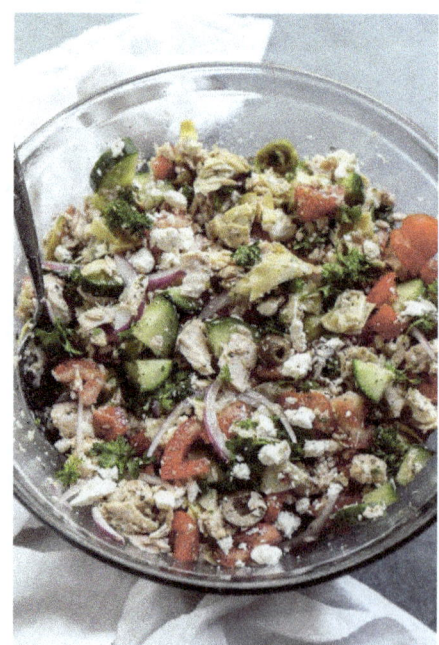

CILANTRO-LIME STEAK SALAD

Prep:
20 mins
Cook:
6 mins
Additional:
10 mins
Total:
36 mins
Servings:
4
Yield:
4 servings

INGREDIENTS:

Dressing:

2 teaspoons seeded and minced jalapeno pepper (Optional)
1 clove garlic
¾ teaspoon minced fresh ginger
⅓ cup lime juice
¼ cup packed cilantro leaves
2 tablespoons honey
2 teaspoons balsamic vinegar
½ teaspoon salt, or to taste
⅓ cup extra-virgin olive oil

Salad:

1 pound flat iron steak
salt and ground black pepper to taste
1 cup corn kernels
1 cup chopped yellow bell pepper
½ cup thinly sliced red onion
1 plum tomato, diced
½ jalapeno pepper, thinly sliced (Optional)
8 cups torn romaine lettuce
½ cup crumbled feta cheese
1 cup tortilla chips, or to taste

DIRECTIONS:

1
To make the dressing, blend jalapeno, garlic,
and ginger in a blender until finely chopped.
Add lime juice, cilantro, honey, balsamic,
and salt; pulse to blend.
With blender running, drizzle in
oil until well incorporated.

2
Preheat oven broiler. Season steak
with salt and black pepper,
then transfer to a foil-lined baking sheet.

3

Broil 4 inches from heat until
an instant-read thermometer inserted
into the center registers
135 degrees F (57 degrees C) for medium-rare,
3 to 4 minutes per side. Let rest about 10 minutes, then thinly slice
against the grain.

4

Stir together corn, bell pepper, red onion,
tomato, and jalapeno (if using) in a bowl.

5

Divide lettuce among 4 plates;
drizzle each with about 2 tablespoons dressing.
Top with steak slices, then with corn mixture.
Sprinkle with feta and garnish with chips.

NUTRITION FACTS:

575 calories; protein 29.9g; carbohydrates 32.1g; fat 38.1g;

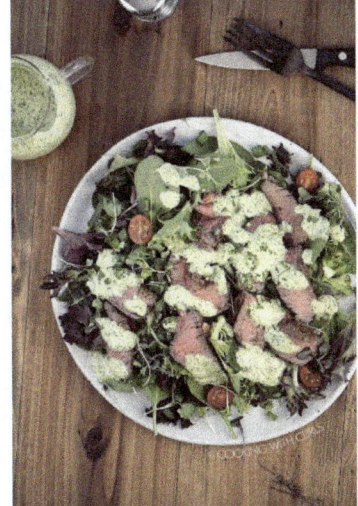

CORNUCOPIA SALAD

Prep:
20 mins
Cook:
5 mins
Additional:
15 mins
Total:
40 mins
Servings:
8
Yield:
8 servings

INGREDIENTS:

¼ cup sliced almonds
1 tablespoon white sugar
1 head red leaf lettuce, torn
3 green onions, chopped
1 Granny Smith apple, cored and chopped
1 avocado - peeled, pitted, and chopped
½ cup dried cranberries
¼ cup crumbled blue cheese

Dressing:

2 tablespoons red wine vinegar
2 teaspoons white sugar
salt and pepper to taste
¼ cup vegetable oil

DIRECTIONS:

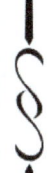

1

Place the almonds and 1 tablespoon of sugar in a small skillet over medium-low heat, and cook and stir until the sugar melts and the almonds brown, watching carefully to avoid burning. Remove from heat and allow to cool.

2

In a large salad bowl, mix the lettuce, green onions, apple, avocado, dried cranberries, blue cheese, and cooked almonds.

3

Whisk together the vinegar, 2 teaspoons of sugar, and salt and pepper in a bowl, and stir in the vegetable oil. Pour the dressing over the salad, and gently toss to combine.

NUTRITION FACTS:

181 calories; protein 2.6g; carbohydrates 15.4g; fat 13.3g;

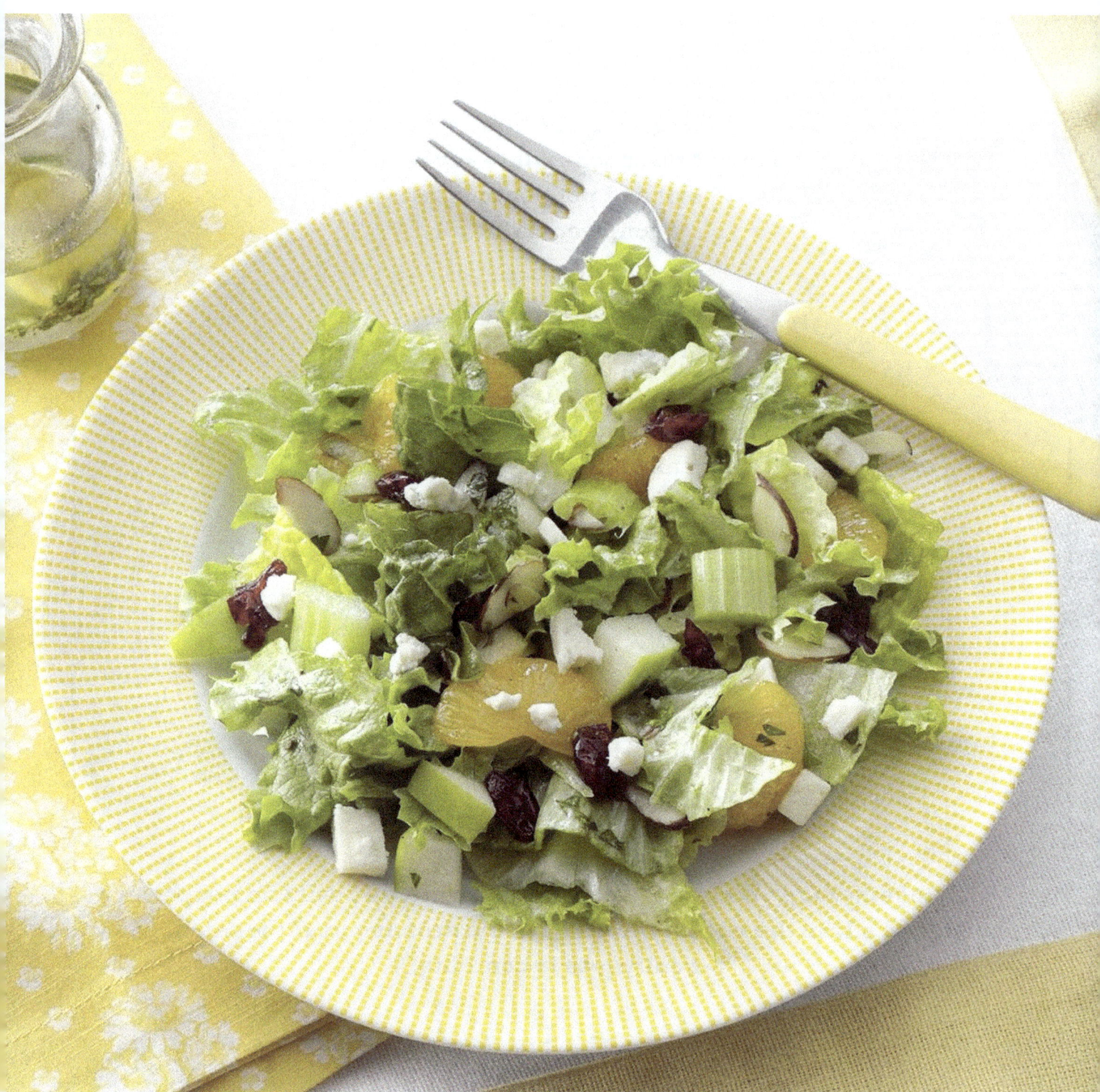

ROQUEFORT PEAR SALAD

Prep:
20 mins
Cook:
10 mins
Total:
30 mins
Servings:
6
Yield:
6 Servings

INGREDIENTS:

1 head leaf lettuce, torn into bite-size pieces
3 pears - peeled, cored and chopped
5 ounces Roquefort cheese, crumbled
3 tablespoons red wine vinegar
1 ½ teaspoons white sugar
1 ½ teaspoons prepared mustard
1 clove garlic, chopped
½ teaspoon salt
fresh ground black pepper to taste
1 avocado - peeled, pitted, and diced
½ cup thinly sliced green onions
¼ cup white sugar
½ cup pecans
⅓ cup olive oil

DIRECTIONS:

1
In a skillet over medium heat,
stir 1/4 cup of sugar together with the pecans.
Continue stirring gently
until sugar has melted and caramelized the pecans.
Carefully transfer nuts onto waxed paper.
Allow to cool, and break into pieces.

2
For the dressing, blend oil,
vinegar, 1 1/2 teaspoons sugar, mustard,
chopped garlic, salt, and pepper.

3
In a large serving bowl, layer lettuce, pears,
blue cheese, avocado, and green onions.
Pour dressing over salad,
sprinkle with pecans, and serve.

NUTRITION FACTS:

426 calories; protein 8g; carbohydrates 33.1g; fat 31.6g;
cholesterol 21.3mg;

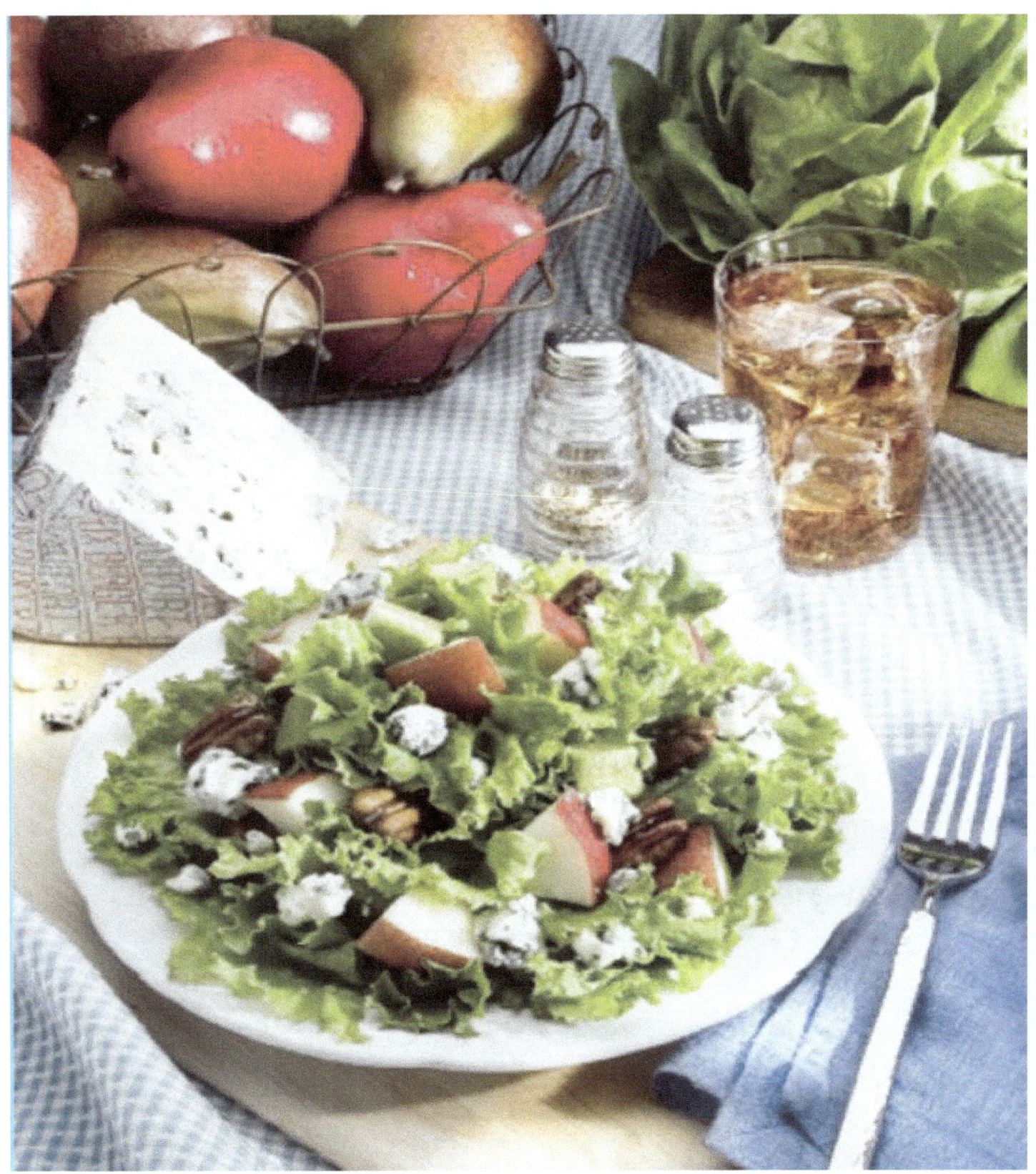

CELERY SALAD WITH SHERRY VINAIGRETTE

Prep:
15 mins
Total:
15 mins
Servings:
4
Yield:
4 servings

INGREDIENTS:

5 tablespoons soybean oil (vegetable oil)
2 tablespoons sherry vinegar
1 small shallot, minced
⅛ teaspoon Dijon mustard
salt to taste
white pepper to taste
1 bunch celery, chopped
1 (12 ounce) can whole kernel corn, drained
1 head leaf lettuce - rinsed, dried, and torn into bite-sized pieces
¼ cup garden cress, or more to taste

DIRECTIONS:

1

Combine celery, corn, lettuce,
and garden cress in a bowl.

2

Mix together oil, sherry vinegar, shallot,
mustard, salt, and pepper in a bowl.
Pour vinaigrette over salad and mix well.

NUTRITION FACTS:

259 calories; protein 4.4g; carbohydrates 23.3g; fat 18.2g;

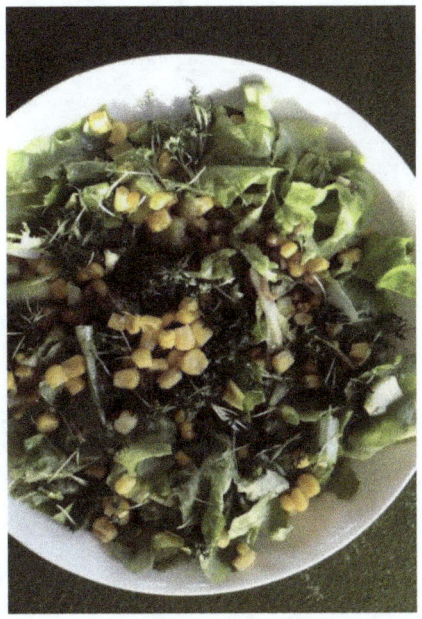

TSIMMES SALAD

Prep:
10 mins
Total:
10 mins
Servings:
2
Yield:
2 servings

INGREDIENTS:

2 medium carrots, peeled and chopped
4 plums, cut into small pieces
1 scallion, chopped

DIRECTIONS:

1
In a bowl, stir together carrots, plums, and scallion.

NUTRITION FACTS:

88 calories; protein 1.6g; carbohydrates 21.5g; fat 0.5g; sodium 43.3mg.

GRILLED EGGPLANT AND ASPARAGUS SALAD

Prep:
10 mins
Cook:
10 mins
Total:
20 mins
Servings:
4
Yield:
4 servings

INGREDIENTS:

2 tablespoons balsamic vinegar
salt and ground black pepper to taste
6 cups chopped romaine lettuce
2 cups chopped endive
2 tablespoons shredded Parmesan cheese, or more to taste
32 asparagus spears, trimmed
2 small Italian eggplants, cut into 1/2-inch thick spears
4 tomatoes, sliced
½ teaspoon salt, or as needed
3 tablespoons olive oil

DIRECTIONS:

1

Preheat grill for medium heat and lightly oil the grate.

2

Toss asparagus, eggplant,
and tomatoes with about 1/2 teaspoon salt.

3

Arrange vegetables on the preheated grill;
cook until tender, 5 to 7 minutes per side.

4

Whisk olive oil and vinegar
in a bowl until smooth;
season to taste with salt and black pepper.
Toss romaine,
endive, and dressing together in a large bowl.

5

Serve grilled vegetables
atop the dressed lettuce mixture;
sprinkle with Parmesan cheese.

NUTRITION FACTS:

195 calories; protein 7.1g; carbohydrates 20.5g; fat 11.7g;
cholesterol 2.2mg;

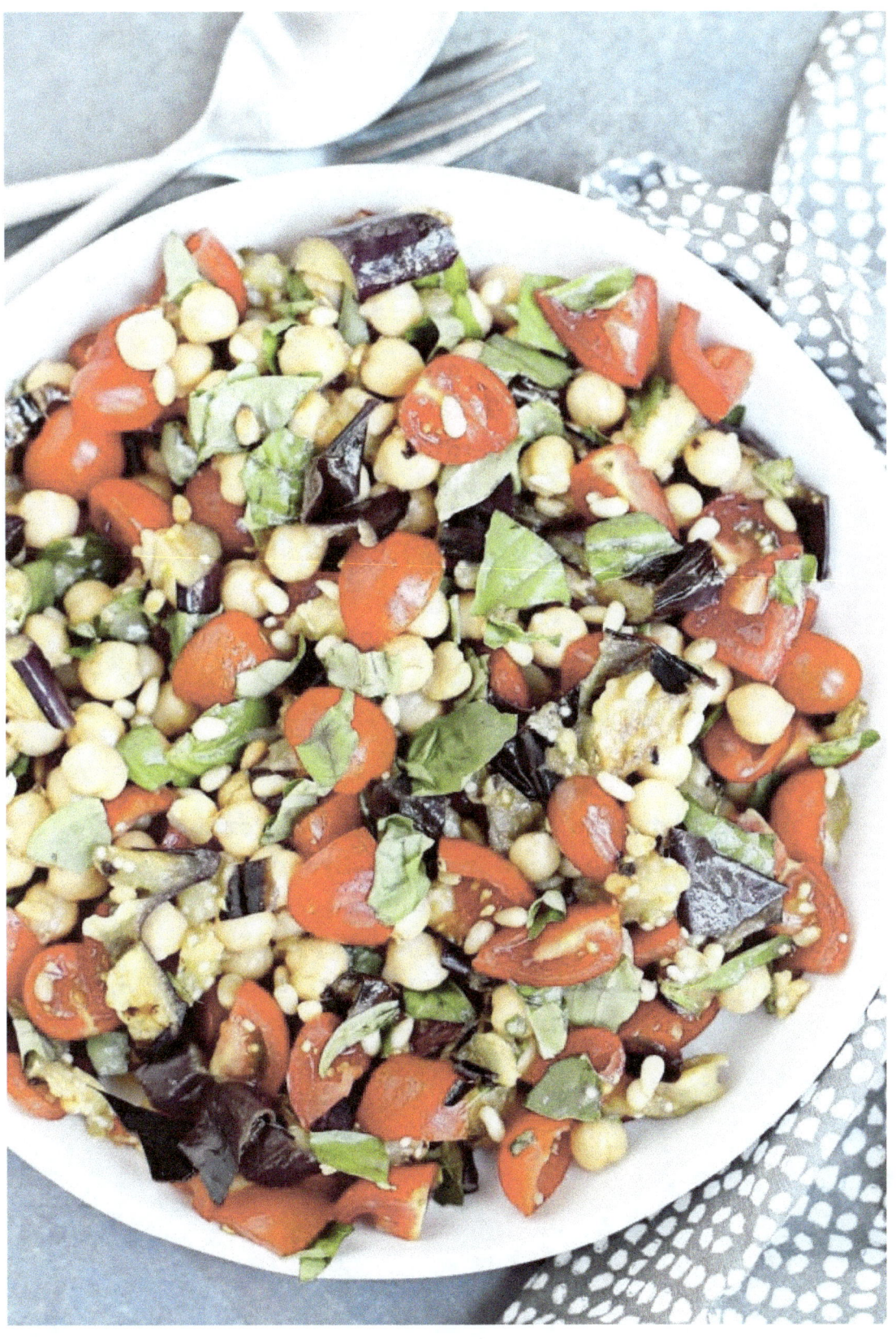

SPINACH, BACON, AND MUSHROOM SALAD

Prep:
15 mins
Cook:
10 mins
Total:
25 mins
Servings:
6
Yield:
6 servings

INGREDIENTS:

4 slices bacon
12 ounces fresh spinach leaves, torn
¾ cup sliced fresh mushrooms
¾ cup croutons
4 hard-cooked eggs, chopped
1 pinch ground black pepper, to taste
¾ cup ranch salad dressing

DIRECTIONS:

1

Fry the bacon in a large, deep skillet over medium-high heat until crisp, about 10 minutes. Drain the bacon slices on a paper towel-lined plate; crumble once cool enough to handle.

2

Toss crumbled bacon, spinach, and mushrooms together in a salad bowl; top with croutons and eggs. Season the salad with black pepper and drizzle with ranch dressing.

NUTRITION FACTS:

266 calories; protein 9.2g; carbohydrates 6.3g; fat 22.8g; cholesterol 156.1mg;

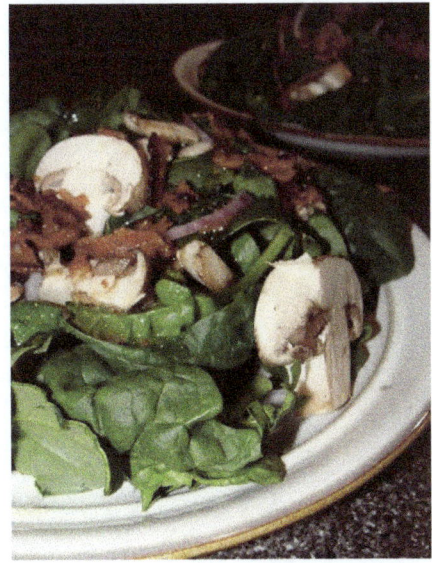

CHAPTER 3: POULTRY RECIPES

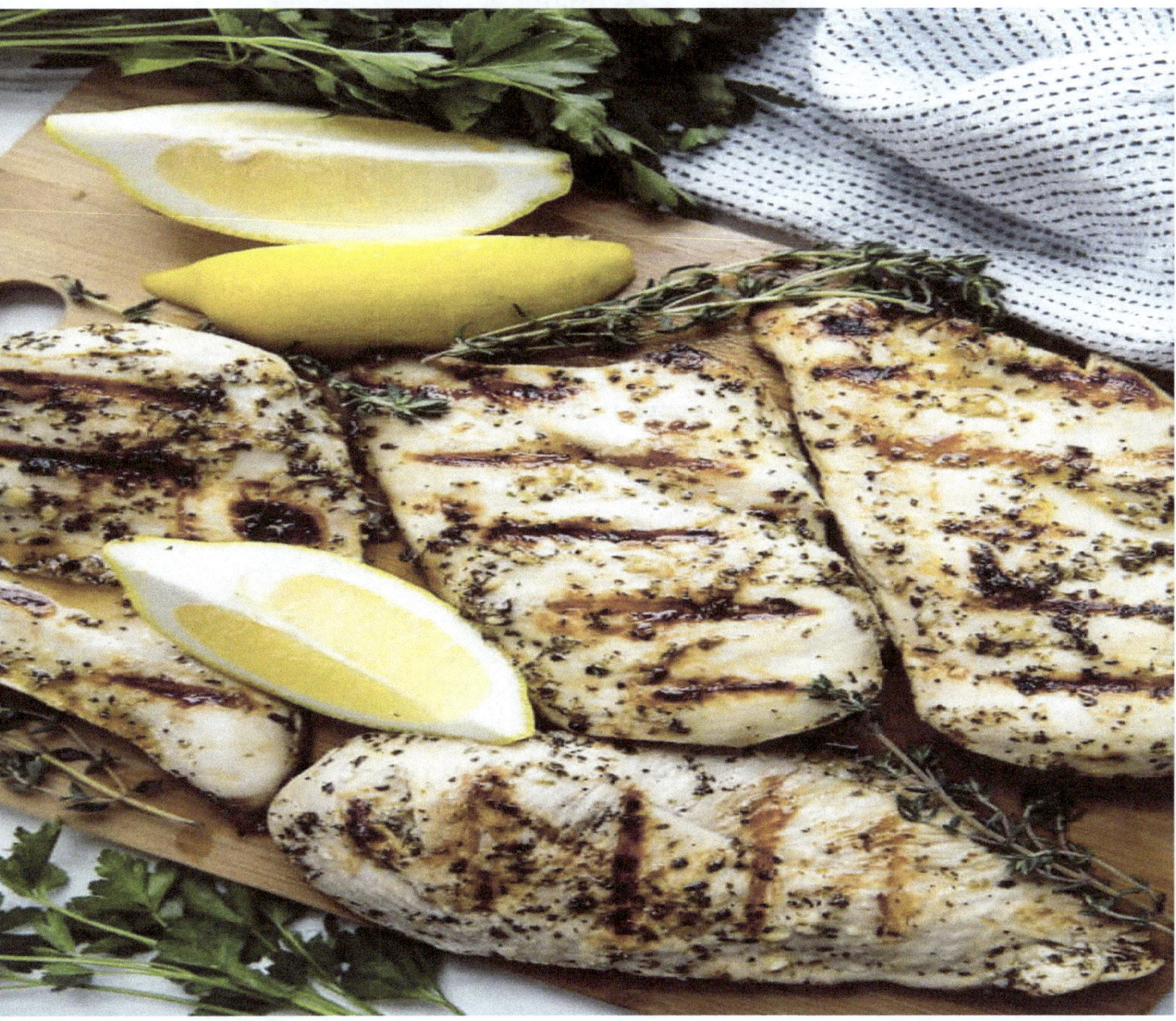

SPICY HOT CHICKEN LEGS

Prep:
5 mins
Cook:
3 hrs
Total:
3 hrs 5 mins
Servings:
6
Yield:
6 servings

INGREDIENTS:

½ teaspoon garlic powder
½ teaspoon onion powder
salt and pepper to taste
1 ½ cups blue cheese salad dressing
12 chicken drumsticks
1 (5 ounce) bottle hot red pepper sauce
¼ cup butter, cubed

DIRECTIONS:

1
Place the drumsticks in a slow cooker,
and sprinkle evenly with pieces of butter.
Pour the hot sauce over the chicken,
then season with garlic powder,
onion powder, salt and pepper.
Cover, and cook on High for 3 hours,
or until tender.
Serve chicken legs with blue cheese dressing on the side.

NUTRITION FACTS:

685 calories; protein 41.4g; carbohydrates 5g; fat 55.6g; cholesterol 158.8mg;

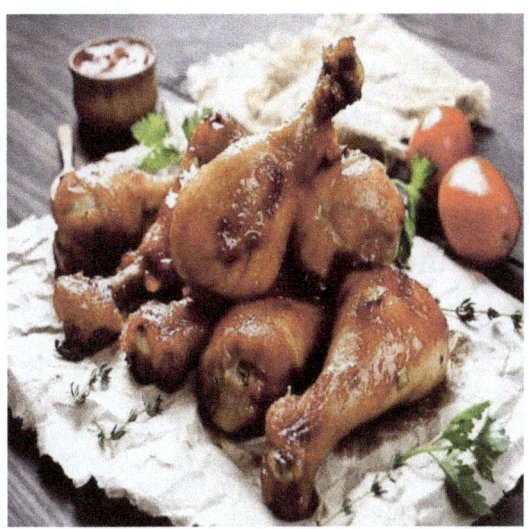

CHICKEN NAPA CABBAGE WRAPS

Prep:
20 mins
Total:
20 mins
Servings:
6
Yield:
6 wraps

INGREDIENTS:

1 tablespoon sliced green onion
3 teaspoons mustard
6 (8 inch) flour tortillas
½ pound diced cooked chicken
1 ½ cups shredded napa cabbage
½ (8 ounce) package cream cheese
½ (8 ounce) container sour cream
6 tablespoons shredded Cheddar cheese

DIRECTIONS:

1
Combine cream cheese, sour cream, Cheddar cheese, green onion, and mustard in a bowl; stir well. Spread 2 tablespoons of the mixture over each tortilla. Top each tortilla with 1/4 cup chicken and 1/4 cup cabbage. Roll up and serve.

NUTRITION FACTS:

396 calories; protein 18.3g; carbohydrates 30g; fat 22.3g;

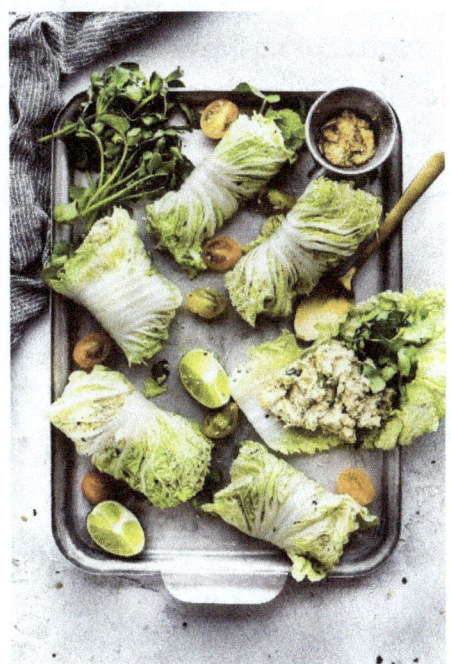

TURKEY WRAPS

Prep:
20 mins
Total:
20 mins
Servings:
6
Yield:
6 wraps

INGREDIENTS:

12 slices thinly sliced deli turkey
¾ cup shredded Swiss cheese
1 large tomato, seeded and diced
1 large avocado, sliced
6 slices bacon, cooked and crumbled
1 (8 ounce) package cream cheese with chives
2 tablespoons Dijon mustard
6 (8 inch) whole wheat tortillas
1 ½ cups finely shredded iceberg lettuce

DIRECTIONS:

1

Mix together the cream cheese and Dijon mustard until smooth. Spread each tortilla with about 2 tablespoons of the cream cheese mixture, spreading to within 1/4 inch of the edge of the tortillas.

2

Arrange about 1/4 cup of shredded lettuce on each tortilla, and press the lettuce down into the cream cheese mixture. Place 2 turkey slices per tortilla over the lettuce, and sprinkle with 2 tablespoons of shredded Swiss cheese. Top each tortilla evenly with tomato, avocado slices, and crumbled bacon.

3

Roll each tortilla up tightly, and cut in half across the middle with a slightly diagonal cut.

NUTRITION FACTS:

457 calories; protein 24.2g; carbohydrates 37.1g; fat 28g; cholesterol 78.4mg;

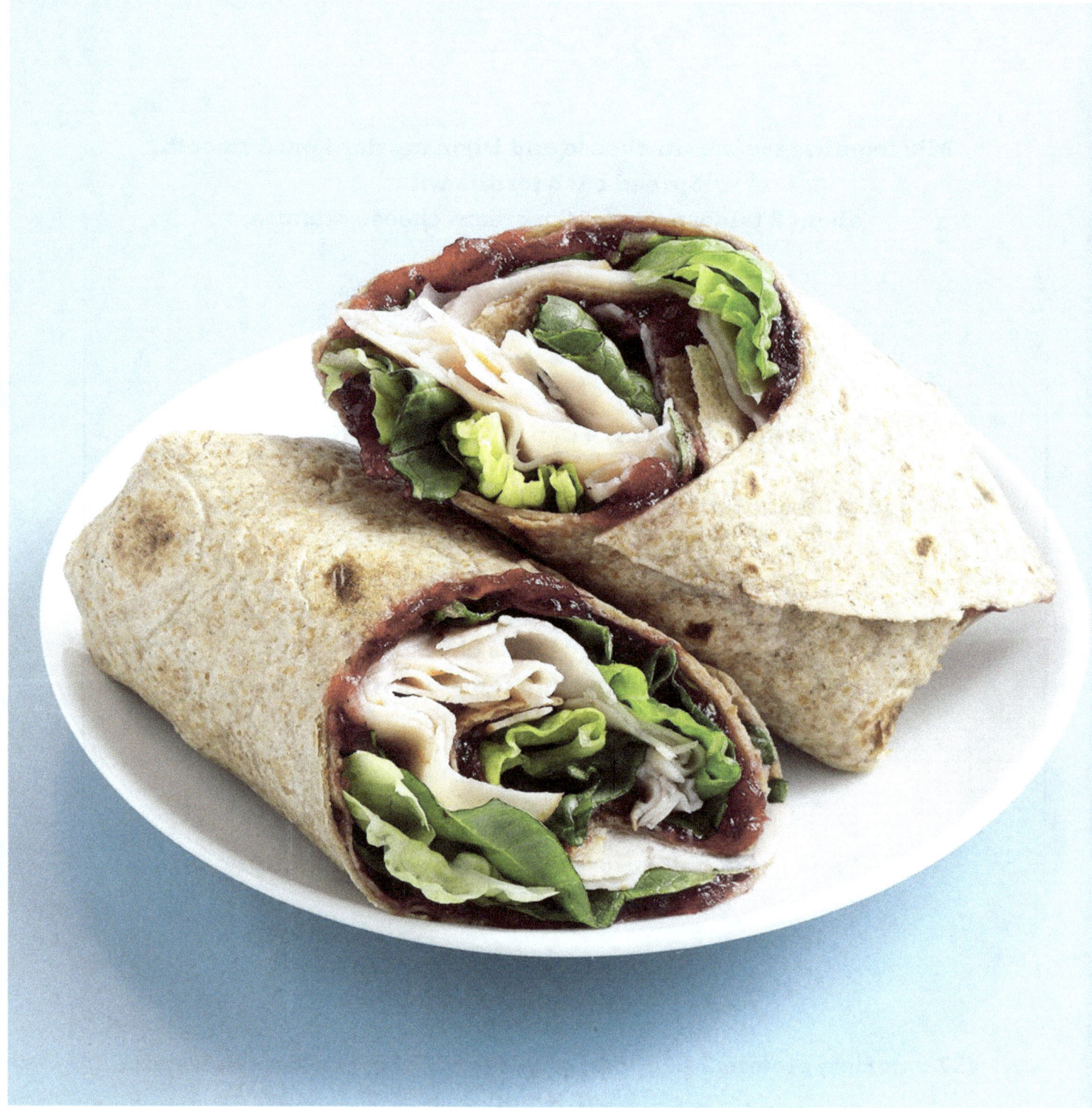

CHICKEN WITH ARTICHOKES AND GOAT CHEESE

Prep:
30 mins
Cook:
55 mins
Total:
1 hr 25 mins
Servings:
4
Yield:
4 servings

INGREDIENTS:

1 cup fresh pearl onions, peeled
½ teaspoon dried thyme
¼ teaspoon salt
¼ teaspoon ground black pepper
3 ounces soft goat cheese, sliced into 4 pieces
2 tablespoons olive oil
4 skinless, boneless chicken breast halves
4 cups chicken stock
1 (9 ounce) package frozen artichoke hearts, thawed
2 tablespoons cornstarch

DIRECTIONS:

1

Heat olive oil in a skillet over medium heat and cook chicken breast halves until browned on both sides, 5 to 8 minutes per side. Pour in chicken stock, artichoke hearts, pearl onions, thyme, salt, and black pepper and bring to a boil. Reduce heat to low and simmer until stock is reduced and onions and artichokes are tender, about 45 minutes; turn chicken breasts over in the skillet after 20 minutes.

2

Place a goat cheese slice on each chicken breast; cover skillet and let goat cheese melt. Place chicken breasts onto a serving platter. Spoon about 3 tablespoons liquid from skillet into a small bowl and whisk in cornstarch until smooth; stir cornstarch mixture into skillet and cook until sauce has thickened, about 1 minute. Serve pan sauce with chicken breasts.

NUTRITION FACTS:

353 calories; protein 32.4g; carbohydrates 17.5g; fat 16.7g; cholesterol 88.9mg;

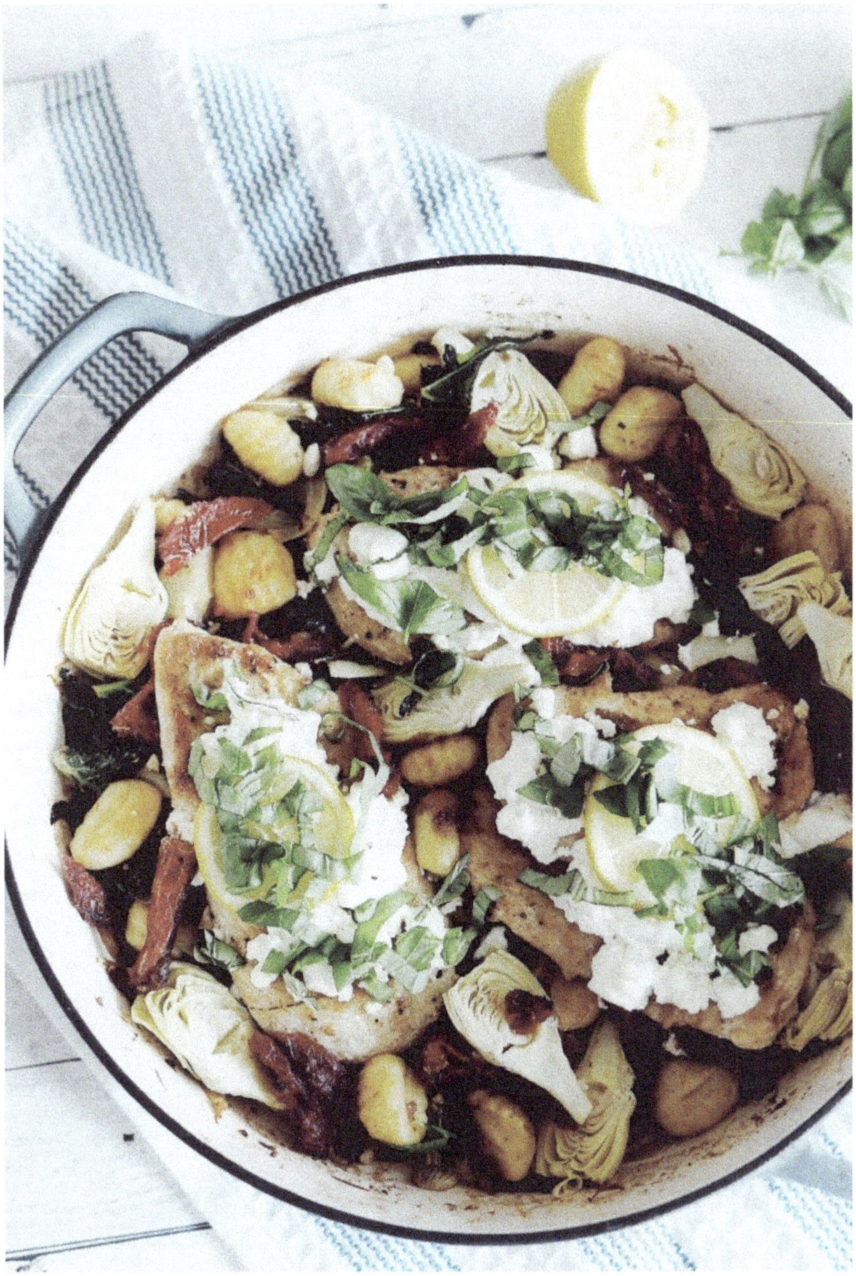

HONEY-GARLIC CHICKEN THIGHS

Servings:
8
Yield:
8 servings

INGREDIENTS:

½ cup soy sauce
1 pinch onion powder, or to taste
1 pinch garlic powder, or to taste
¼ cup chopped fresh cilantro
8 (5 ounce) boneless chicken thighs
salt and ground black pepper to taste
2 tablespoons olive oil, or as needed
½ medium onion, finely chopped
7 cloves garlic, chopped, or to taste
1 cup honey

DIRECTIONS:

1

Season the chicken on both sides with salt and pepper.

2

Cover the bottom of a cast iron skillet with olive oil and bring to medium-high heat. Add chicken and brown on one side, 3 to 5 minutes. Flip chicken, and add onion and garlic; continue to cook until chicken is mostly (but not fully) cooked and onion and garlic are soft, 5 to 7 minutes more. Remove chicken to a plate.

3

Add honey, soy sauce, onion powder, garlic powder, and onion powder to the skillet. Stir and scrape the bottom of the pan with a wooden spoon to get the garlic and onion to mix with the liquid.

4

Put chicken back into the pan, cover,
and reduce heat to medium.
Cook until no longer pink in the center and juices run clear,
about 10 more minutes, turning once halfway through.
An instant-read thermometer inserted
into the center of a thigh should
read at least 165 degrees F (74 degrees C).

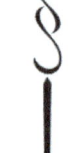

5

Place on a serving tray and drizzle liquid
from the pan on top. Sprinkle
with chopped cilantro before serving

NUTRITION FACTS:

368 calories; protein 25.3g; carbohydrates 37.9g; fat 13.4g;

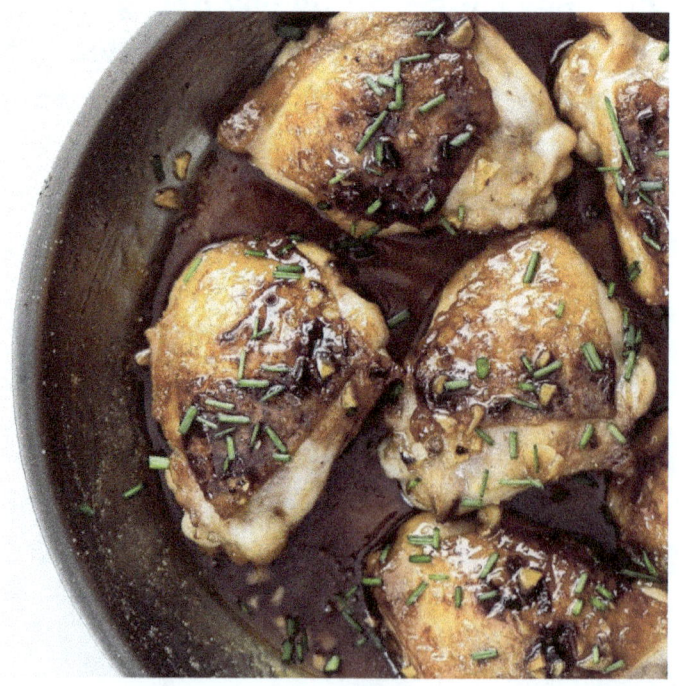

TENDER BREADED TURKEY CUTLETS

Prep:
10 mins
Cook:
15 mins
Total:
25 mins
Servings:
4
Yield:
4 servings

INGREDIENTS:

4 turkey breast cutlets, 1/4 inch thick
½ cup fat free sour cream
1 tablespoon extra virgin olive oil
1 cup Italian seasoned dry bread crumbs
¼ cup grated Parmesan cheese

DIRECTIONS:

1

Mix the bread crumbs and cheese in a shallow dish.
Spread both sides of turkey with sour
cream and press into the
bread crumb mixture to coat.

2

Heat the oil in a skillet over medium heat.
Place turkey in the skillet
and cook 5 to 7 minutes on each side,
until lightly browned and cooked through.

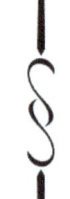

NUTRITION FACTS:

397 calories; protein 53.1g; carbohydrates 24.8g; fat 7.9g;
cholesterol 133.5mg;

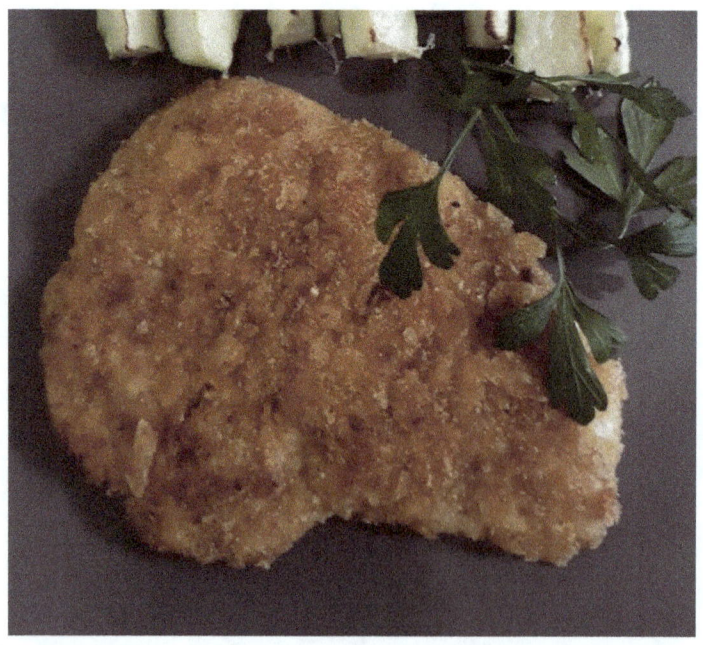

FANTASTIC CREAMY ALMOND CHICKEN BAKE

Prep:
15 mins
Cook:
40 mins
Total:
55 mins
Servings:
4
Yield:
4 servings

INGREDIENTS:

bread crumbs
2 cups ranch dressing
1 (10.75 ounce) can cream of celery soup
1 cup shredded mozzarella cheese
½ cup slivered almonds
1 cup shredded Cheddar cheese
1 cup crushed potato chips, or to taste
4 skinless, boneless chicken breast halves
2 tablespoons olive oil, or more to taste
2 cups cooked white rice

DIRECTIONS:

1

Preheat oven to 400 degrees F (200 degrees C).

2

Spread bread crumbs into a wide, shallow bowl. Press chicken breast halves into bread crumbs to coat. Gently pat chicken to let any loose crumbs fall away. Place coated breasts onto a plate while breading the rest; do not stack.

3

Heat olive oil in a skillet over medium-high heat. Cook chicken in hot oil to brown completely, 3 to 5 minutes per side.

4

Spread rice into the bottom of a 13x9-inch baking dish. Arrange browned chicken breasts atop the rice.

5
Mix ranch dressing,
celery soup, mozzarella cheese,
and almonds together in a bowl;
pour over the chicken and rice,
assuring the chicken is covered completely.
Sprinkle Cheddar cheese over the ranch
dressing mixture and top
with crushed potato chips.

6
Bake in preheated oven until golden brown
on top and the chicken is no longer pink in the center,
30 to 40 minutes.
An instant-read thermometer inserted
into the center should
read at least 165 degrees F (74 degrees C).

NUTRITION FACTS:

protein 52.7g; carbohydrates 65.9g; fat 105.6g;

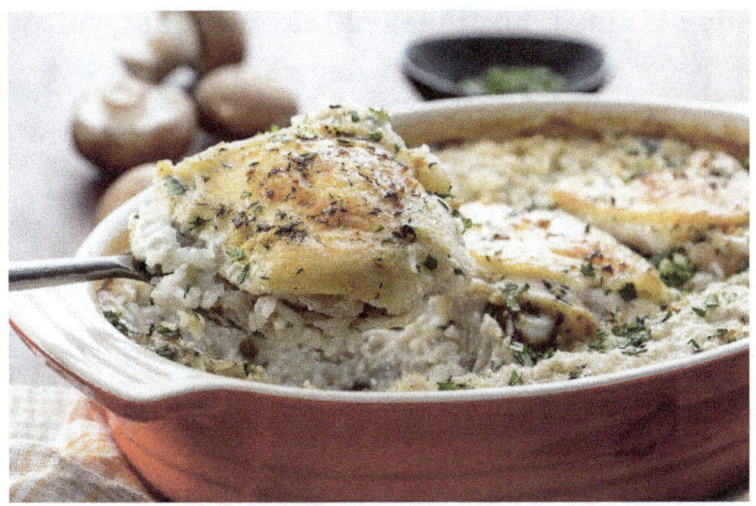

FIVE SPICE CHICKEN

Prep:
10 mins
Cook:
6 mins
Additional:
1 hr
Total:
1 hr 16 mins
Servings:
5
Yield:
5 servings

INGREDIENTS:

¼ cup soy sauce
2 tablespoons olive oil
1 teaspoon minced fresh ginger root
2 teaspoons Chinese five-spice powder
1 ½ pounds skinless, boneless chicken breast, thinly sliced
1 tablespoon dry sherry
1 tablespoon orange juice
1 teaspoon minced garlic

DIRECTIONS:

1

Whisk soy sauce, olive oil, sherry, orange juice, garlic, ginger, and Chinese five-spice powder together in a bowl; pour into a resealable plastic bag. Add chicken, coat with the marinade, squeeze bag to remove excess air, and seal the bag. Marinate in the refrigerator at least 1 hour.

2

Preheat grill for medium heat and lightly oil the grate.

3

Remove chicken slices from the marinade; shake to remove excess moisture. Discard remaining marinade.

4

Grill chicken until no longer pink in the center and the juices run clear, about 3 minutes per side.

NUTRITION FACTS:

234 calories; protein 31.4g; carbohydrates 3.3g; fat 9.8g;

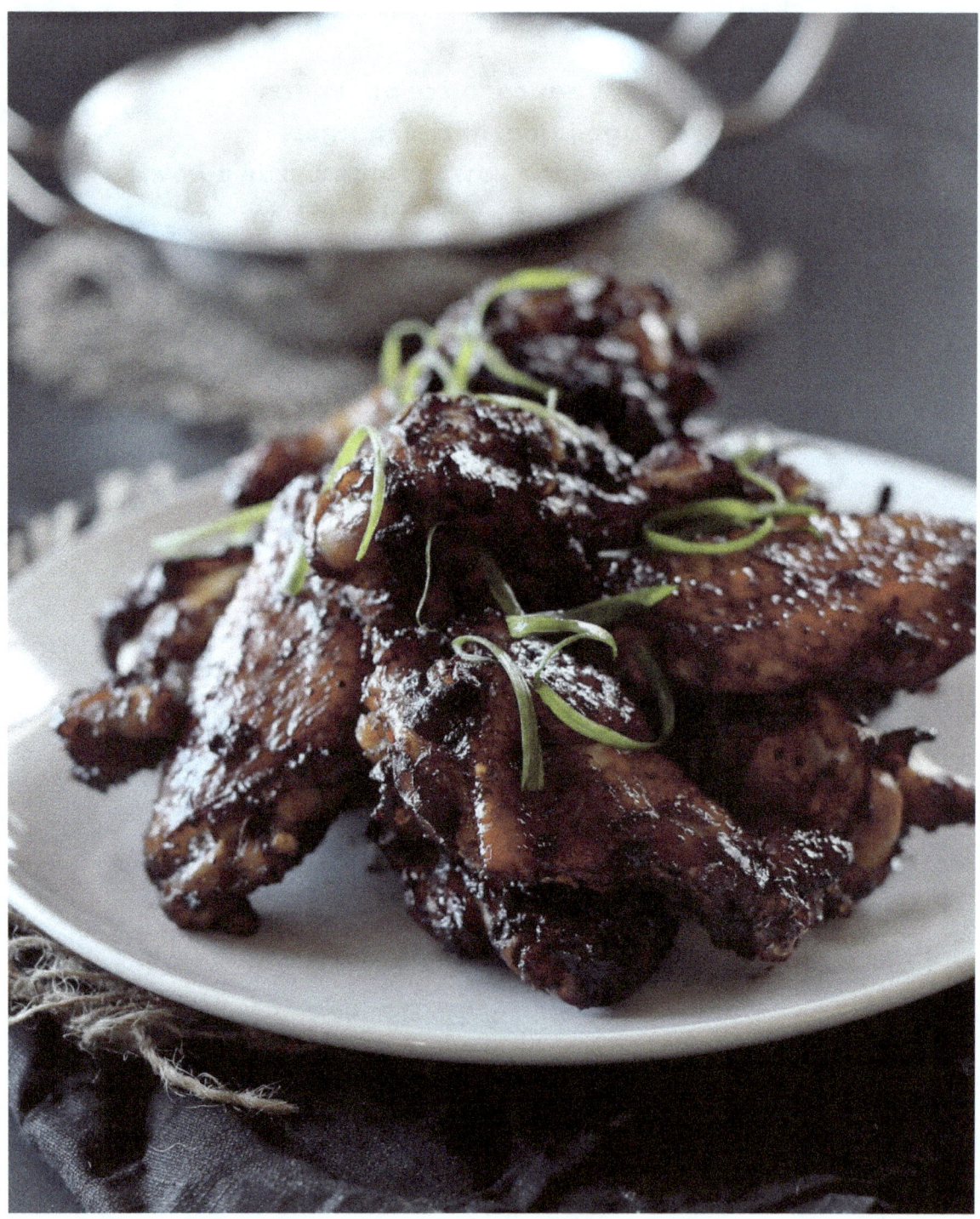

ROASTED ROSEMARY CHICKEN AND VEGETABLES

Servings:
4
Yield:
4 servings

INGREDIENTS:

1 green bell pepper, sliced
1 red bell pepper, sliced
1 small red onion, quartered
3 carrots, cut into 1 inch pieces
1 eggplant, cut into 1/2 inch cubes
⅓ cup olive oil
⅓ cup balsamic vinegar
1 tablespoon dried rosemary
½ teaspoon crushed red pepper flakes
1 clove garlic, minced
4 skinless, boneless chicken breasts

DIRECTIONS:

1

Preheat oven to 400 degrees F (200 degrees C).
Line a cookie sheet with aluminum foil,
and coat with cooking spray.

2

In a large bowl, combine olive oil, balsamic vinegar,
rosemary, red pepper flakes, and garlic.
Place chicken in the bowl, and marinate 5 minutes.
Transfer to a baking dish,
reserving marinade in the bowl.

3

Place green bell pepper, red bell pepper,
red onion, carrots, and eggplant in the marinade,
and toss to coat. Arrange in a single layer
on the prepared cookie sheet.

4

Place the chicken and vegetables in the preheated oven.
Bake chicken for 20 minutes, or until juices run clear.
Bake the vegetables for 35 minutes, or until the edges
of the vegetables brown.

NUTRITION FACTS:

381 calories; protein 27.3g; carbohydrates 21g; fat 21.6g;

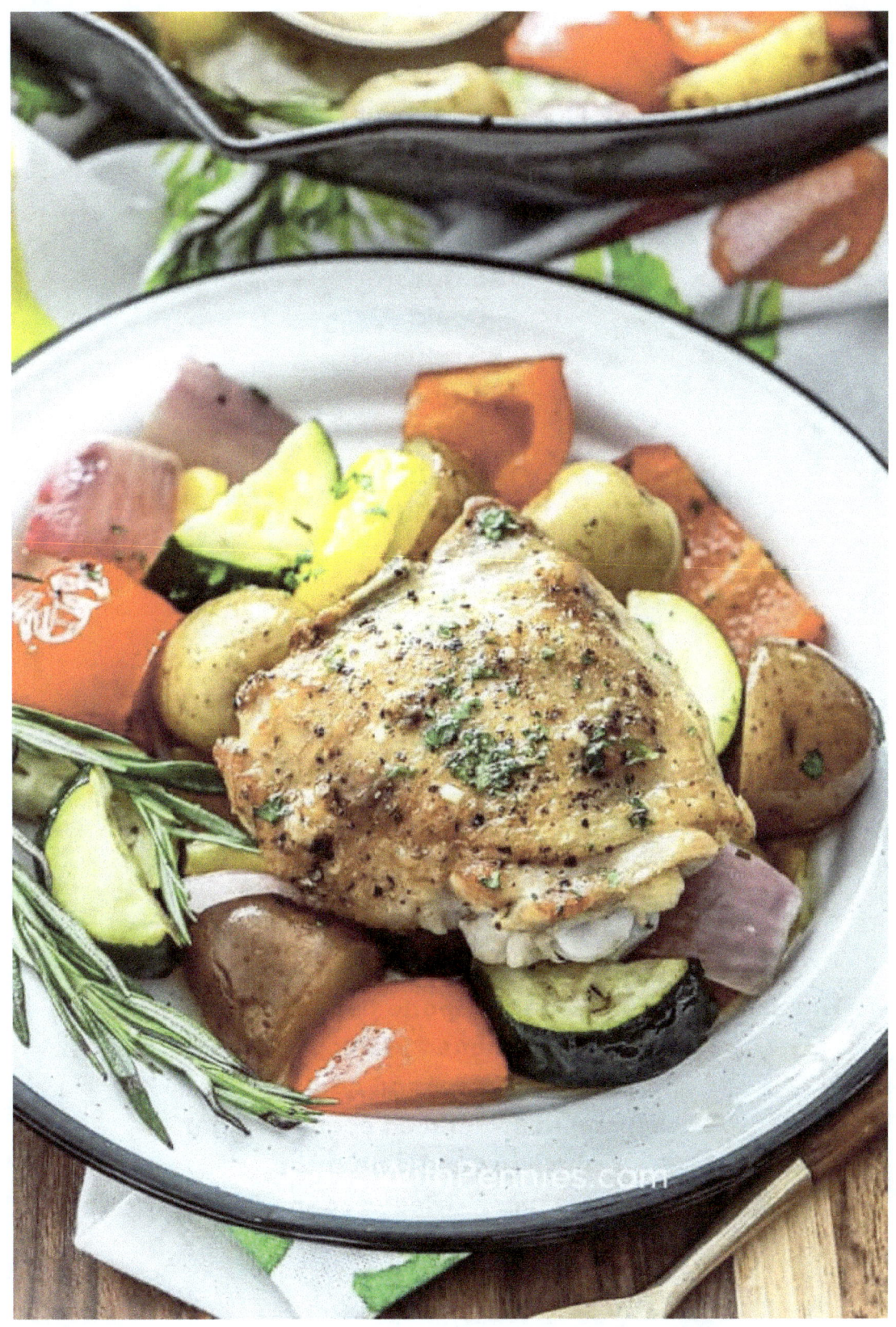

TURKEY CHILI MAC

Prep:
15 mins
Cook:
50 mins
Additional:
5 mins
Total:
1 hr 10 mins
Servings:
6
Yield:
6 servings

INGREDIENTS:

2 tablespoons olive oil
1 medium yellow onion, diced
1 teaspoon salt, or more to taste
2 tablespoons chili powder, or to taste
½ teaspoon ground dried chipotle pepper, or more to taste
1 teaspoon ground black pepper
1 teaspoon ground cumin
1 teaspoon unsweetened cocoa powder
1 pinch ground cinnamon
½ teaspoon dried oregano
3 cloves garlic, minced

4 cups chicken broth, or more as needed
1 (10 ounce) can diced tomatoes with green chile peppers
1 cup tomato sauce
1 pound coarsely chopped leftover turkey
1 (15 ounce) can pinto beans, rinsed and drained
1 cup elbow macaroni
½ cup grated white Cheddar cheese

DIRECTIONS:

1
Heat olive oil in a pot over medium-high heat. Add onion and 1 teaspoon salt; cook, stirring, until it starts to soften and turns translucent, about 5 minutes.

2
While onion cooks, make the spice mixture by combining chili powder, chipotle pepper, cumin, black pepper, cocoa, cinnamon, and oregano in a small bowl.

3
Add garlic and the spice mixture to the onion and cook, stirring, 1 to 2 minutes.

4

Stir in 4 cups chicken broth, diced tomatoes with chiles,
and tomato sauce.
Raise the heat to high and bring to a simmer.
Reduce the heat to medium-low and simmer,
stirring occasionally,
for 15 minutes.

5

Add the leftover turkey meat along
with additional chicken broth if needed, and cook,
stirring occasionally, for another 15 minutes.

6

Taste for salt and other seasonings and adjust as needed.
Raise the heat to high and bring to a boil.
Stir in pinto beans and elbow macaroni
and cover tightly with a lid. Cook, covered,
until the pasta is just barely tender,
about 5 minutes.

7

Turn off the heat, remove the lid, and stir very well.
Cover back up and let sit with the heat off for 5 minutes.
Uncover, stir in Cheddar cheese,
and serve immediately

NUTRITION FACTS:

373 calories; protein 32.2g; carbohydrates 29.9g; fat 13.9g;

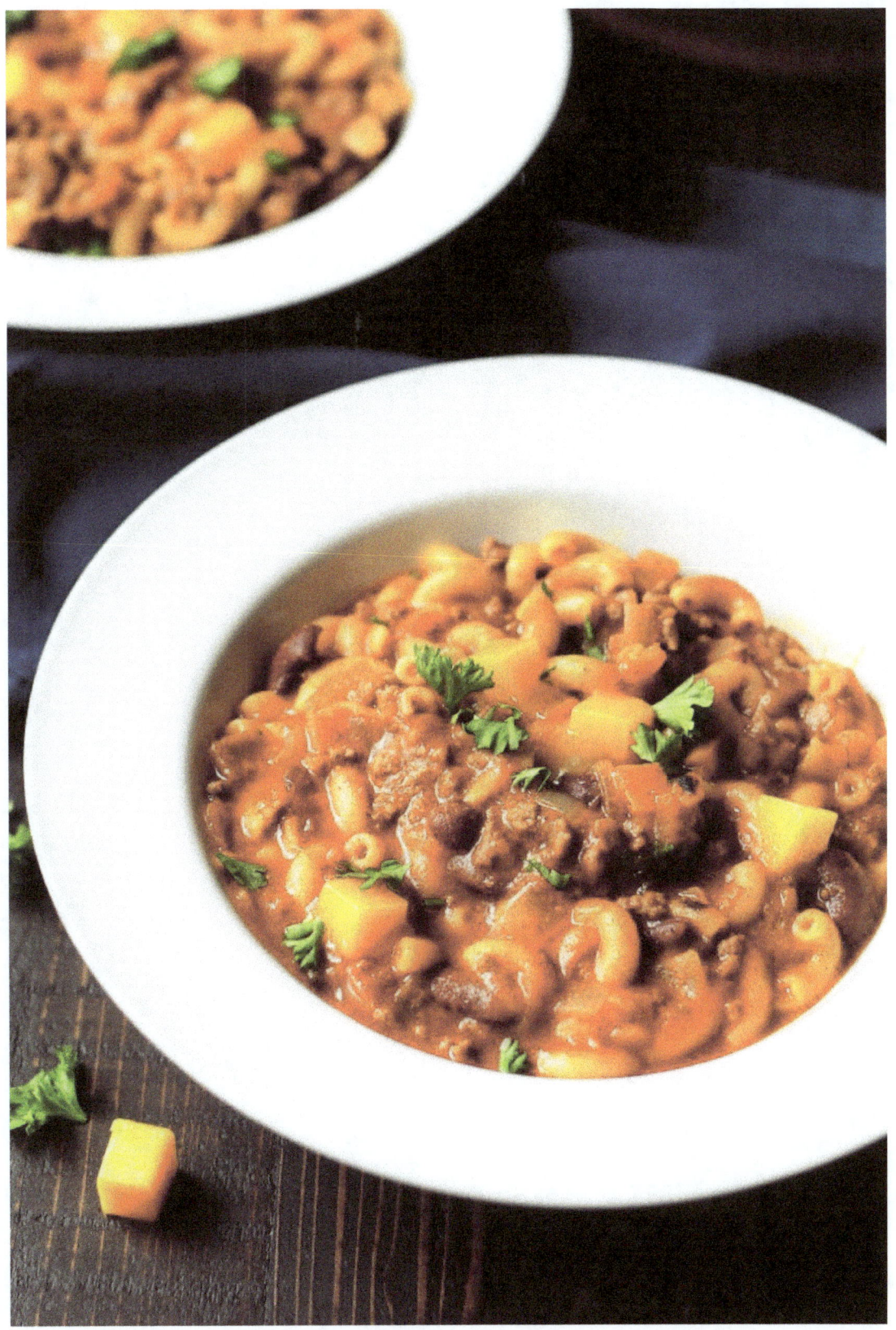

CHAPTER 4: FISH & SEAFOOD RECIPES

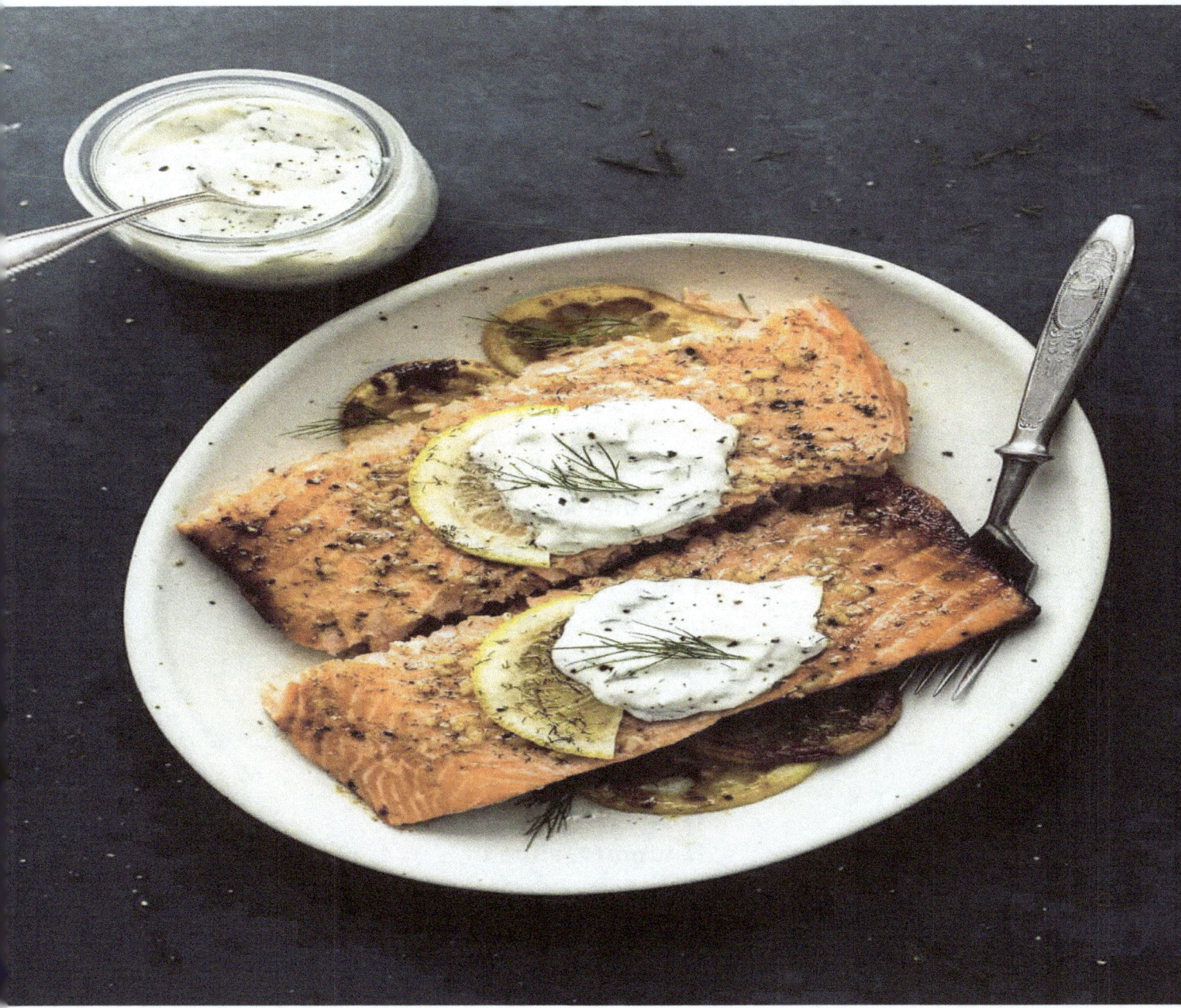

AMAZING TUNA BURGERS

Prep:
22 mins
Cook:
8 mins
Total:
30 mins
Servings:
4
Yield:
4 servings

INGREDIENTS:

1 (5 ounce) can tuna, drained
1 egg
½ cup Italian seasoned bread crumbs
⅓ cup minced onion
¼ cup minced celery
¼ cup mayonnaise
2 tablespoons chili sauce
½ teaspoon dried dill weed
¼ teaspoon salt
⅛ teaspoon ground black pepper
¼ cup minced red bell pepper
4 hamburger buns
1 tomato, sliced
4 leaves of lettuce (Optional)
1 dash hot pepper sauce
1 dash Worcestershire sauce

DIRECTIONS:

1

Combine tuna, egg, bread crumbs, onion, celery, red bell pepper, mayonnaise, hot chili sauce, chili sauce, dill, salt, pepper, hot pepper sauce and Worcestershire sauce. Mix well. Shape into 4 patties (mixture will be very soft and delicate). Refrigerate for 30 minutes to make the patties easier to handle, if desired.

2

Coat a non-stick skillet with cooking spray; fry tuna patties for about 3 to 4 minutes per side, or until cooked through. These are fragile, so be careful when turning them.

3

Serve on buns with tomato slices and lettuce leaves, if desired.

NUTRITION FACTS:

353 calories; protein 16.4g; carbohydrates 36.6g; fat 15.6g;

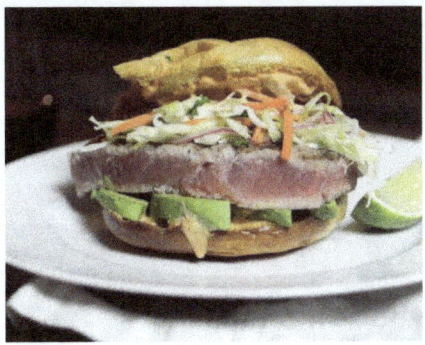

SALMON WITH DILL

Prep:
5 mins
Cook:
25 mins
Total:
30 mins
Servings:
4
Yield:
4 servings

INGREDIENTS:

1 teaspoon onion powder
1 teaspoon dried dill weed
2 tablespoons butter
1 pound salmon fillets or steaks
¼ teaspoon salt
½ teaspoon ground black pepper

DIRECTIONS:

1

Preheat oven to 400 degrees F (200 degrees C).

2

Rinse salmon, and arrange
in a 9x13 inch baking dish.
Sprinkle salt, pepper, onion powder,
and dill over the fish.
Place pieces of butter evenly over the fish.

3

Bake in preheated oven for 20 to 25 minutes.
Salmon is done
when it flakes easily with a fork.

NUTRITION FACTS:

262 calories; protein 22.8g; carbohydrates 0.7g; fat 18.1g;

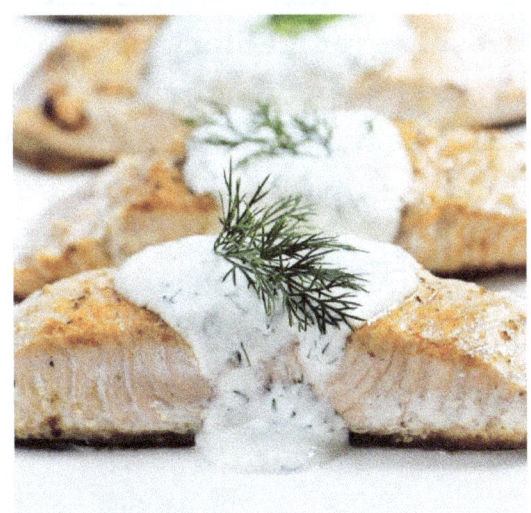

GARLICKY SHRIMP SCAMPI

Prep:
15 mins
Cook:
6 mins
Total:
21 mins
Servings:
6
Yield:
6 servings

INGREDIENTS:

6 tablespoons unsalted butter, softened
¼ cup olive oil
1 tablespoon minced garlic
1 tablespoon minced shallots
2 tablespoons minced fresh chives
salt and freshly ground black pepper to taste
½ teaspoon paprika
2 pounds large shrimp - peeled and deveined

DIRECTIONS:

1

Preheat grill for high heat.

2

In a large bowl, mix together softened butter, olive oil, garlic, shallots, chives, salt, pepper, and paprika; add the shrimp, and toss to coat.

3

Lightly oil grill grate. Cook the shrimp as close to the flame as possible for 2 to 3 minutes per side, or until opaque.

NUTRITION FACTS:

303 calories; protein 25g; carbohydrates 0.9g; fat 21.8g;

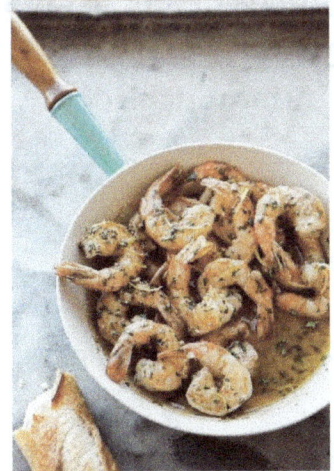

GRILLED PESTO SHRIMP SKEWERS

Prep:
10 mins
Cook:
10 mins
Additional:
30 mins
Total:
50 mins
Servings:
8
Yield:
8 skewers

INGREDIENTS:

8 wooden skewers
1 pound large shrimp, peeled and deveined
3 ounces pesto, divided
3 tablespoons chopped fresh basil
1 lemon, sliced

DIRECTIONS:

1
Fill a dish with water
and soak skewers for 30 minutes.

2
Preheat an outdoor grill for medium
heat and lightly oil the grate.

3
Thread shrimp onto skewers;
place on a large serving dish.
Brush skewers with 1 ounce pesto.

4
Grill shrimp skewers on the preheated grill
until they are bright pink on the outside and the meat is opaque,
about 4 minutes per side.
Brush cooked shrimp with 1 ounce pesto.
Sprinkle with basil and serve
with remaining pesto and lemon slices.

NUTRITION FACTS:

103 calories; protein 11.5g; carbohydrates 2.3g; fat 5.7g;

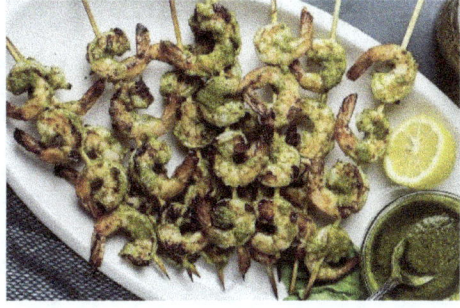

STUFFED SOLE WITH IMITATION CRAB

Prep:
25 mins
Cook:
25 mins
Total:
50 mins
Servings:
4
Yield:
4 servings

INGREDIENTS:

1 tablespoon dried minced onion
¾ teaspoon dried parsley
1 pinch cayenne pepper
salt and ground black pepper to taste
4 (4 ounce) sole fillets
¼ cup bread crumbs
6 ounces imitation crabmeat, flaked
⅓ cup diced red bell pepper
⅓ cup diced celery
⅓ cup shredded mozzarella cheese
2 tablespoons creamy salad dressing

DIRECTIONS:

1

Preheat an oven to 450 degrees F (230 degrees C).

2

Place the imitation crabmeat, bell pepper,
celery, and mozzarella cheese into a mixing bowl.
Gently stir in the creamy salad dressing,
dried onion, parsley, and cayenne pepper.
Season to taste with salt and pepper.
Place a sole fillet onto your work surface,
and place 1/4 of the crab mixture onto one end.
Roll the sole over the filling, and secure with a toothpick.
Repeat with the remaining fillets,
and place into a close-fitting baking dish, side by side.
Cover with aluminum foil

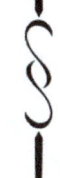

3

Bake in the top third of the preheated oven for 15 minutes.
Remove the aluminum foil,
and sprinkle evenly with breadcrumbs.
Return to the oven,
and continue baking until the fish is flaky,
and the filling is hot, 10 to 15 minutes more.

NUTRITION FACTS:

223 calories; protein 27.8g; carbohydrates 14.2g; fat 5.3g;

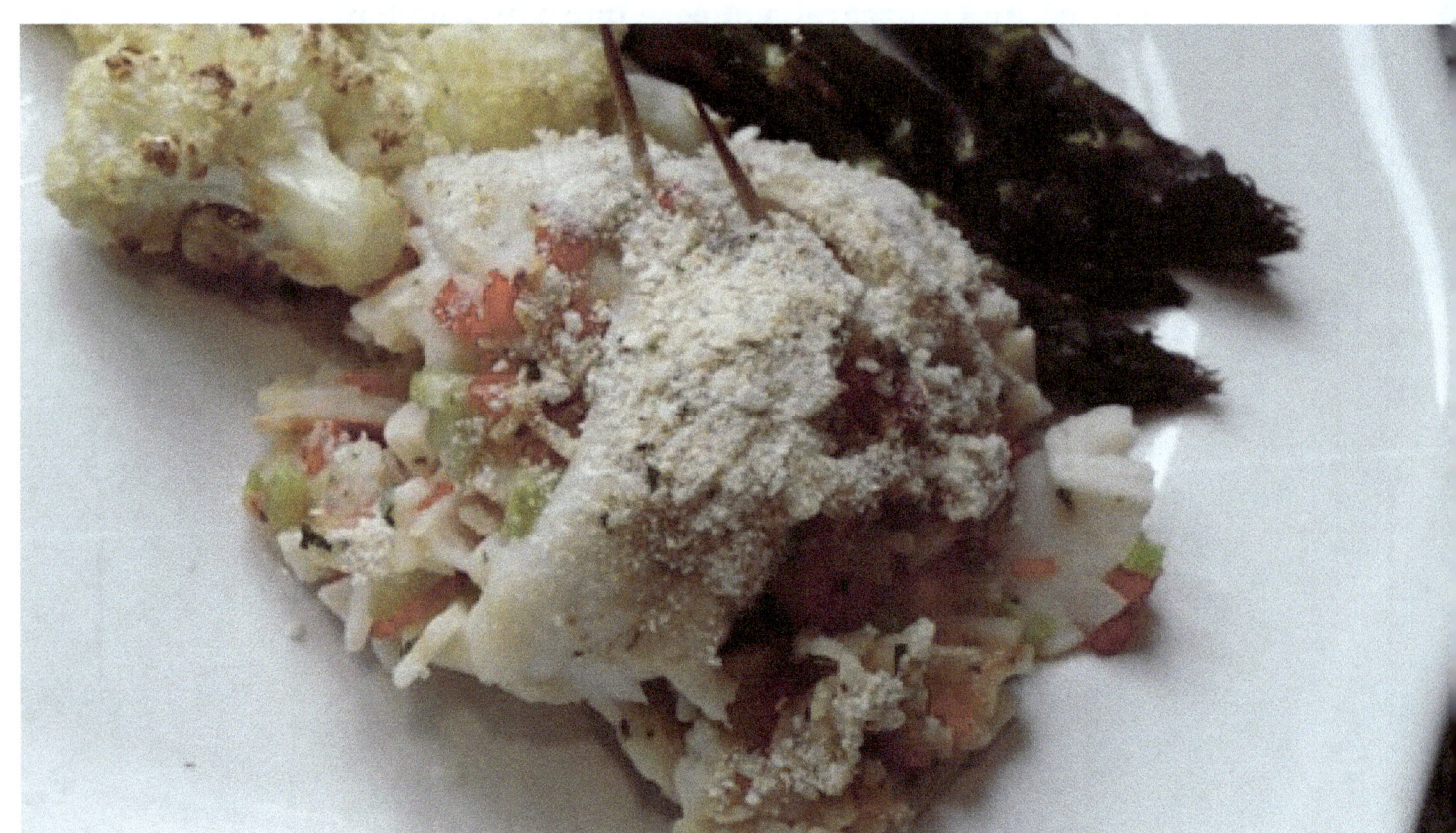

CHAPTER 5: SOUP & STEW RECIPES

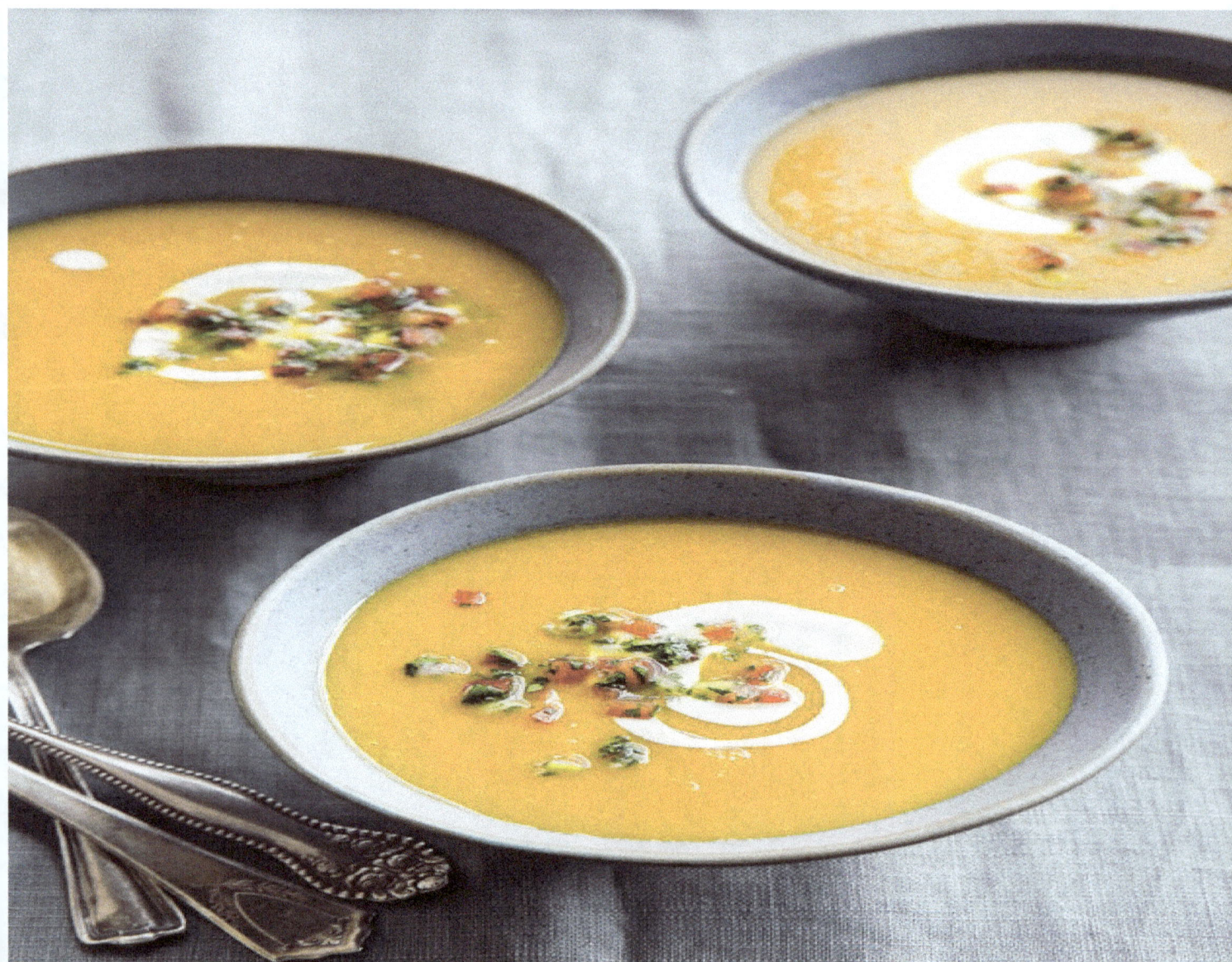

ASPARAGUS SOUP

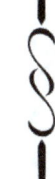

Prep:
20 mins
Cook:
15 mins
Total:
35 mins
Servings:
4
Yield:
4 servings

INGREDIENTS:

1 onion, chopped
2 tablespoons butter
1 pound fresh asparagus, trimmed and coarsely chopped
1 cup vegetable broth
1 dash garlic powder
1 dash white pepper
1 cup 1% milk

DIRECTIONS:

1

Microwave onion and butter
on HIGH for 2 minutes.
Add asparagus, vegetable broth,
garlic powder and white pepper.
Microwave, covered,
on HIGH for 10 to 12 minutes.
Puree in blender.

2

Return mixture to microwave safe dish,
stir in milk and microwave
until heated through.

DIRECTIONS:

119 calories; protein 5.2g; carbohydrates 11.2g; fat 6.8g;

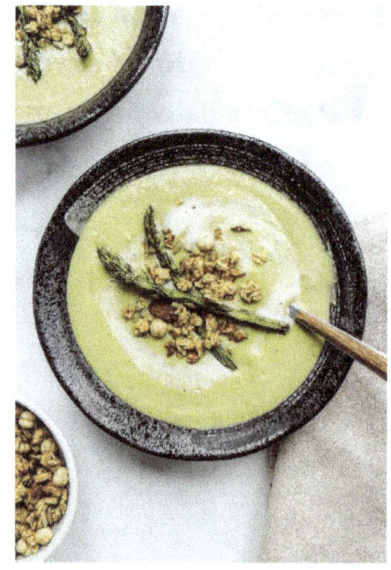

CHICKPEA SOUP

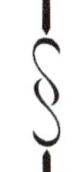

Prep:
25 mins
Cook:
35 mins
Total:
1 hr
Servings:
6
Yield:
6 servings

INGREDIENTS:

2 tablespoons olive oil
1 onion, chopped
2 cloves garlic, minced
2 cups peeled and chopped sweet potatoes
3 cups chicken broth
1 bay leaf
1 teaspoon dried basil
½ teaspoon dried thyme
¼ teaspoon paprika
1 tomato, chopped
1 (10 ounce) package frozen mixed vegetables
1 (15 ounce) can garbanzo beans, drained
salt to taste
ground black pepper to taste

DIRECTIONS:

1

In a saucepan, warm oil over moderate heat.
Add onion, garlic, and sweet potatoes;
saute 5 minutes.

2

Stir in broth, bay leaf, basil, thyme, and paprika.
Salt and pepper to taste.
Bring to a boil, and then reduce heat to medium low.
Cover. Simmer until vegetables are tender but not mushy,
about 15 minutes.

3

Stir in tomato, green beans, and chickpeas.
Simmer uncovered until tender,
about 10 minutes more. Serve hot.

NUTRITION FACTS:

198 calories; protein 7.5g; carbohydrates 29.6g; fat 6.1g;

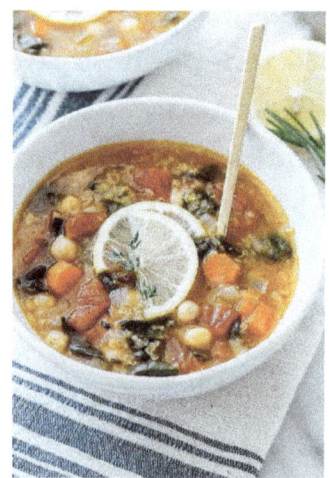

SEAFOOD STEW

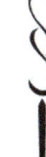

Prep:
30 mins
Cook:
45 mins
Total:
1 hr 15 mins
Servings:
10
Yield:
10 servings

INGREDIENTS:

1 quart milk
1 pint half-and-half
½ cup unsalted butter
1 (750 milliliter) bottle white wine
½ (12 ounce) bottle cocktail sauce
1 tablespoon celery salt
1 tablespoon hot sauce
1 teaspoon prepared horseradish
1 teaspoon Worcestershire sauce
seasoned salt to taste
coarsely ground black pepper to taste
1 pound medium shrimp - peeled and deveined
2 whole crabs - cleaned, cracked, shell removed
3 (8 ounce) cans oysters
paprika to taste

DIRECTIONS:

1

In a large pot over medium heat,
mix the milk,
half-and-half, butter, wine, cocktail sauce,
celery salt, hot sauce, horseradish,
and Worcestershire sauce. Season with seasoned salt,
and pepper.
Cook and stir until heated through.

2

Mix the shrimp,
crab, and oysters into the pot, and continue cooking 30 minutes.
Spoon into bowls
and sprinkle with paprika to serve.

NUTRITION FACTS:

392 calories; protein 23.2g; carbohydrates 15.6g; fat 20.1g;

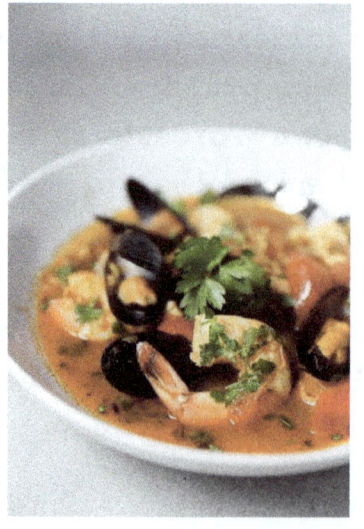

VEGAN CREAM OF ASPARAGUS SOUP

Prep:
15 mins
Cook:
20 mins
Additional:
5 mins
Total:
40 mins
Servings:
4
Yield:
4 servings

INGREDIENTS:

2 tablespoons coconut oil
1 onion, diced
2 cloves garlic, minced
1 ½ teaspoons salt, or more to taste
1 teaspoon finely chopped fresh rosemary
1 teaspoon finely chopped fresh thyme
¼ teaspoon freshly ground black pepper
2 pounds fresh asparagus, trimmed and cut into 2-inch pieces
½ cup unsalted raw cashews
3 ½ cups vegetable broth
1 (14 ounce) can organic coconut milk
1 ½ tablespoons lemon juice

DIRECTIONS:

1
Combine coconut oil and onion in a large
pot over medium heat and cook,
stirring occasionally,
until onion is soft and translucent, about 5 minutes.
Stir in garlic, salt, rosemary, thyme, and pepper;
cook for 1 to 2 minutes.
Add asparagus.
Cook and stir over medium heat for 5 minutes.

2
Reduce heat to medium-low and add cashews,
vegetable broth, and coconut milk.
Bring to a low boil, cover,
and simmer until asparagus is tender,
7 to 10 minutes.
Turn off heat and stir in lemon juice.
Let stand until cooled slightly.

3
Puree asparagus soup using
an immersion blender until smooth.
Garnish with chopped parsley.

NUTRITION FACTS:

434 calories; protein 11.4g; carbohydrates 24.5g; fat 36.1g;

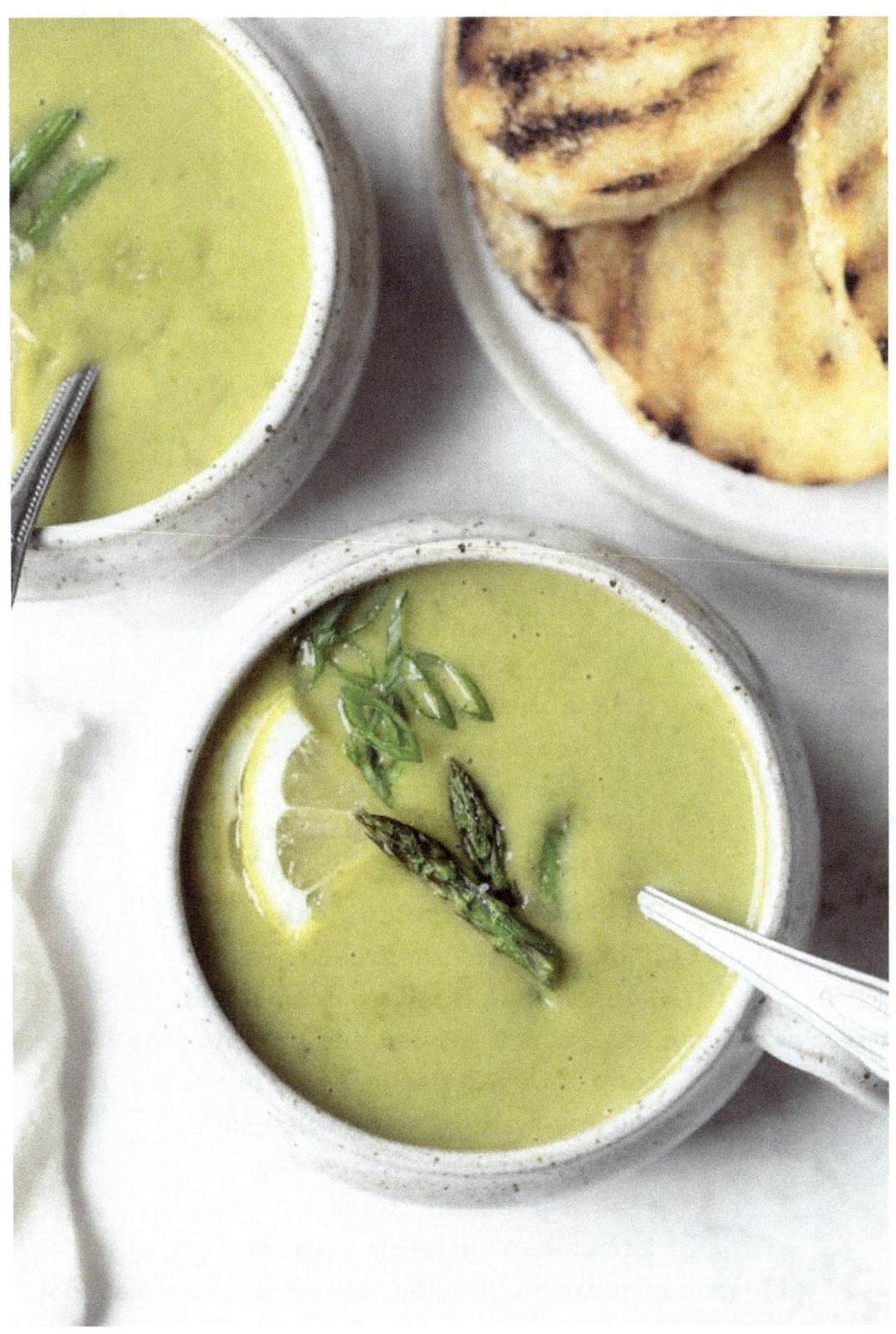

GREEN DETOX SOUP

Prep:
25 mins
Cook:
30 mins
Total:
55 mins
Servings:
10
Yield:
10 servings

INGREDIENTS:

2 tablespoons olive oil
1 ½ cups chopped fennel
1 ⅓ cups sliced leeks
1 ¼ cups chopped celery
2 cloves garlic, smashed
1 (10 ounce) zucchini, cubed
1 (10 ounce) package fresh spinach
½ (12 ounce) bag fresh broccoli florets
6 leaves Tuscan kale, ribs removed and cut into small pieces
¼ cup chopped flat-leaf parsley
4 cups low-sodium vegetable broth
2 cups hot water as needed
1 avocado, diced
1 teaspoon spirulina powder
10 tablespoons gomasio (toasted, crushed sesame seeds)

DIRECTIONS:

1

Heat oil in a Dutch oven over medium heat.
Add fennel, leeks, celery, and garlic cloves
and saute until soft and fragrant, 3 to 5 minutes.
Add zucchini, spinach, broccoli, kale, and parsley;
mix to combine.
Cook until kale and spinach have wilted slightly,
about 3 minutes.

2

Stir in vegetable broth and bring to a boil.
Reduce heat and simmer, covered,
until vegetables are soft, about 15 minutes.
Remove from the heat.
Puree soup with an immersion
blender until smooth,
adding hot water if needed to achieve desired consistency.
Add avocado and spirulina
powder and blend until smooth.

3

Ladle soup into bowls and serve
each with 1 tablespoon gomasio.

NUTRITION FACTS:

147 calories; protein 6.1g; carbohydrates 14.4g; fat 10.6g;

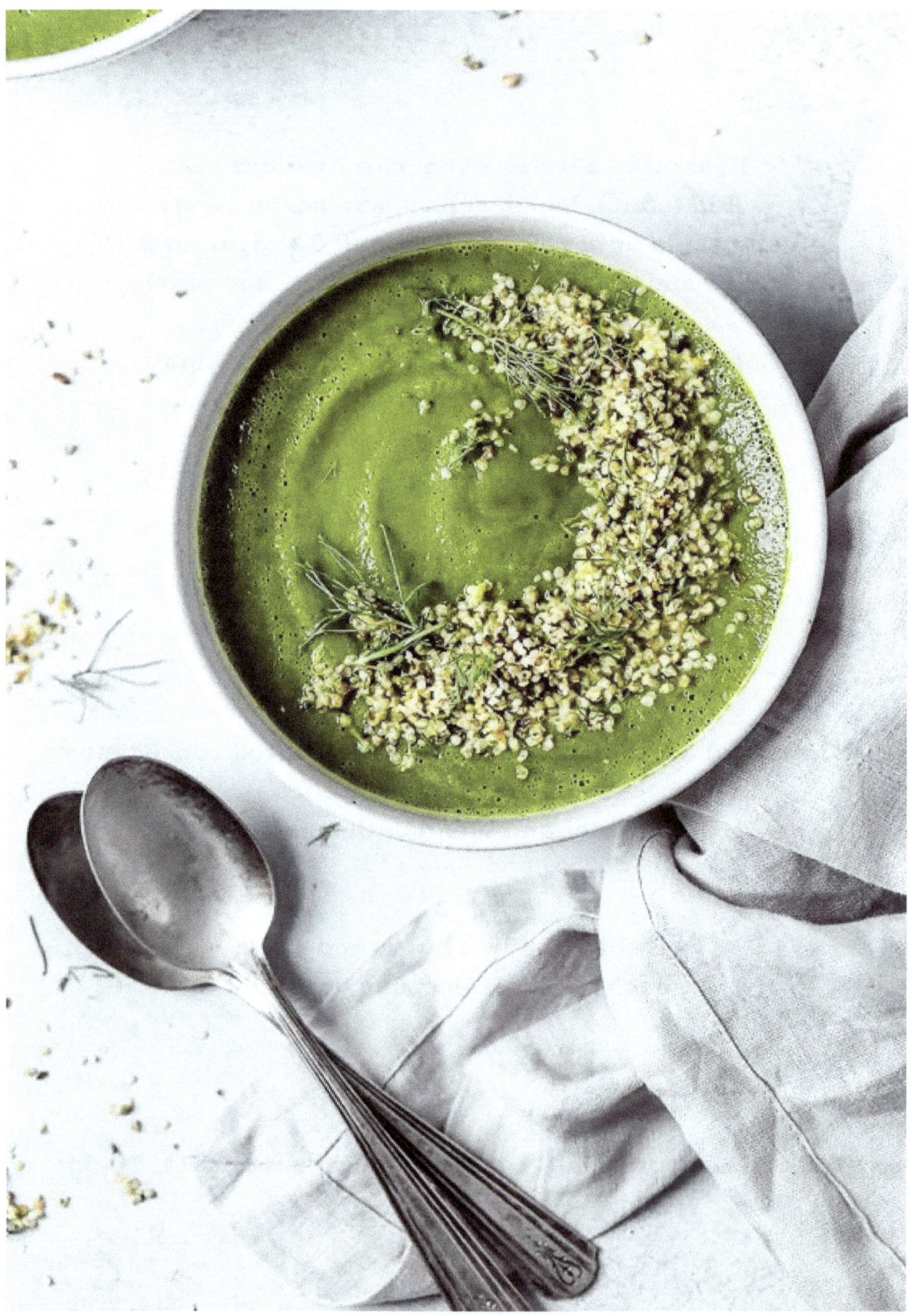

CHAPTER 6: MEAT RECIPES

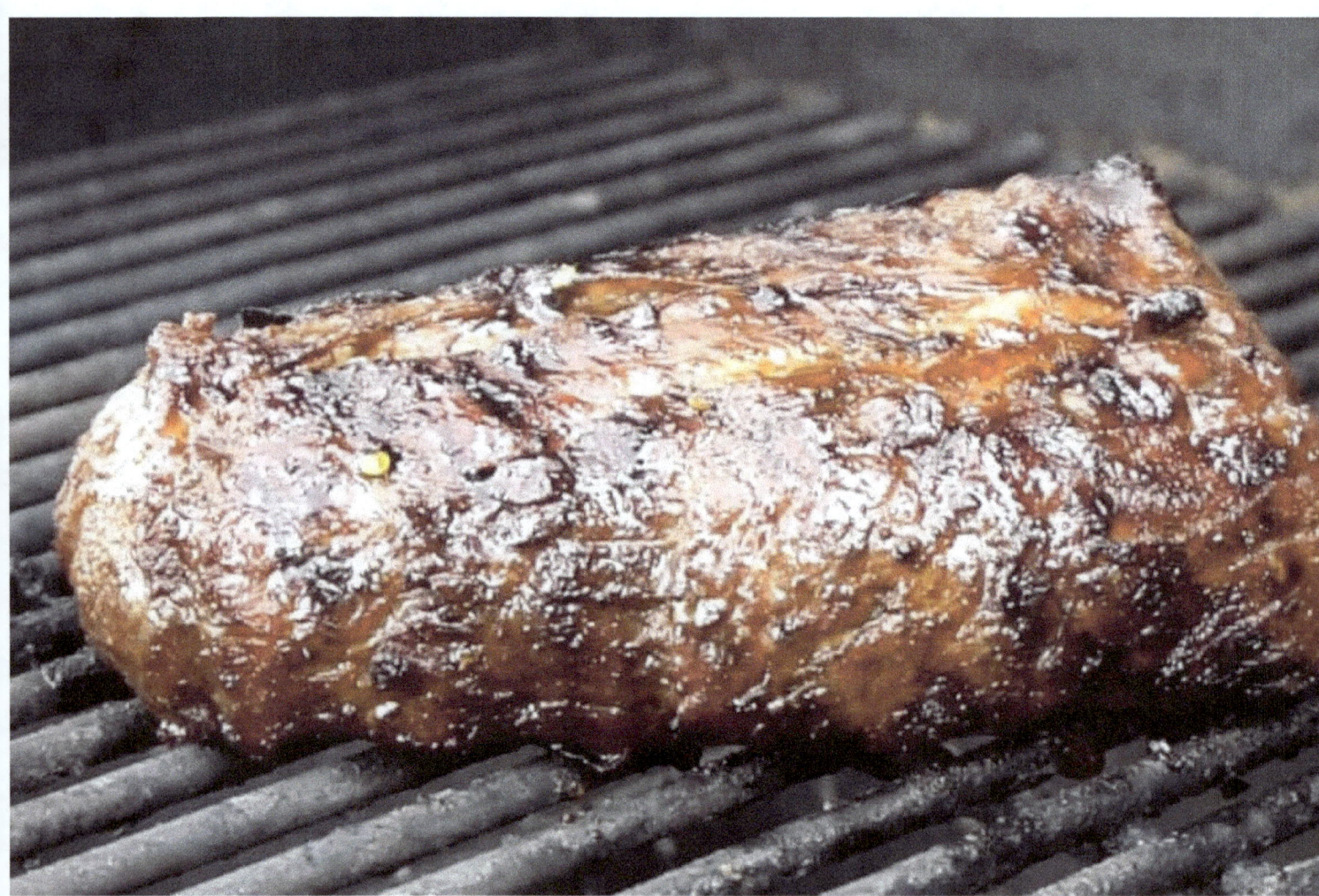

BEEF PEPPER STEAK

Prep:
10 mins
Cook:
20 mins
Additional:
1 hr
Total:
1 hr 30 mins
Servings:
2
Yield:
2 servings

INGREDIENTS:

12 black peppercorns, coarsely ground
2 tablespoons tamari
1 clove garlic, minced
1 pinch white sugar
1 pinch salt
10 ounces beef filet
2 tablespoons butter

DIRECTIONS:

1

In a small, nonporous bowl, combine the peppercorns,
tamari, garlic, sugar and salt.
Add the beef filet and coat well on all sides.
Cover and marinate
in the refrigerator for 1 hour.

2

Melt butter in a medium saucepan over medium high heat.
Place the beef filet in the pan
and saute for 6 to 8 minutes per side,
or until internal temperature reaches
at least 145 degrees F (65 degrees C).

NUTRITION FACTS:

533 calories; protein 27.9g; carbohydrates 5.9g; fat 44.4g

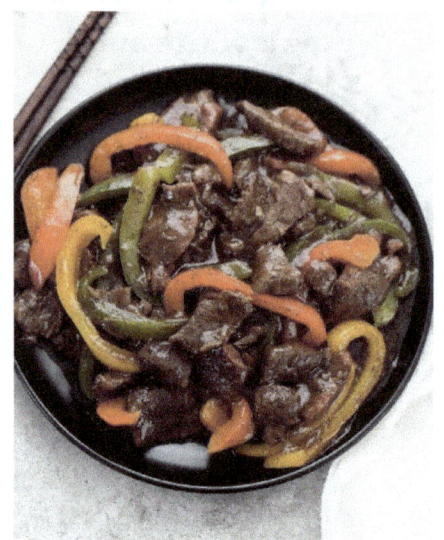

PORK TENDERLOIN WITH TOMATO AND PEPPER SAUCE

Prep:
20 mins
Cook:
1 hr 10 mins
Total:
1 hr 30 mins
Servings:
4
Yield:
4 servings

INGREDIENTS:

2 teaspoons butter
1 teaspoon minced garlic
1 (1 1/2 pound) lean pork tenderloin, cut into thin strips
1 (14.5 ounce) can diced tomatoes and green chiles
1 teaspoon dried basil
1 ½ teaspoons salt
1 ½ teaspoons freshly ground black pepper
½ cup water
1 ½ cups thinly sliced green bell pepper
1 onion, diced

DIRECTIONS:

1

In a large skillet, melt butter over medium-high heat.
Stir garlic into sizzling hot butter,
and then arrange as many
sliced pork tenderloin strips as you can fit into the pan.
Cook, turning occasionally,
until browned on both sides. Remove from pan; set aside.
Repeat with any remaining pork tenderloin strips.

2

Return all pork tenderloin strips to pan.
Stir in tomatoes and season with basil, salt, and pepper.
Cook until mixture comes to a boil,
then reduce heat to low, and cover.

3

Meanwhile, heat water in a nonstick skillet over medium heat.
Cook peppers and onion in boiling-hot water until
vegetables are tender-crisp.
Stir into pork tenderloin and tomatoes.
Continue cooking until
pork tenderloin strips are no longer pink,
about 50 to 60 minutes.

NUTRITION FACTS:

264 calories; protein 36.9g; carbohydrates 9.7g; fat 8.3g;

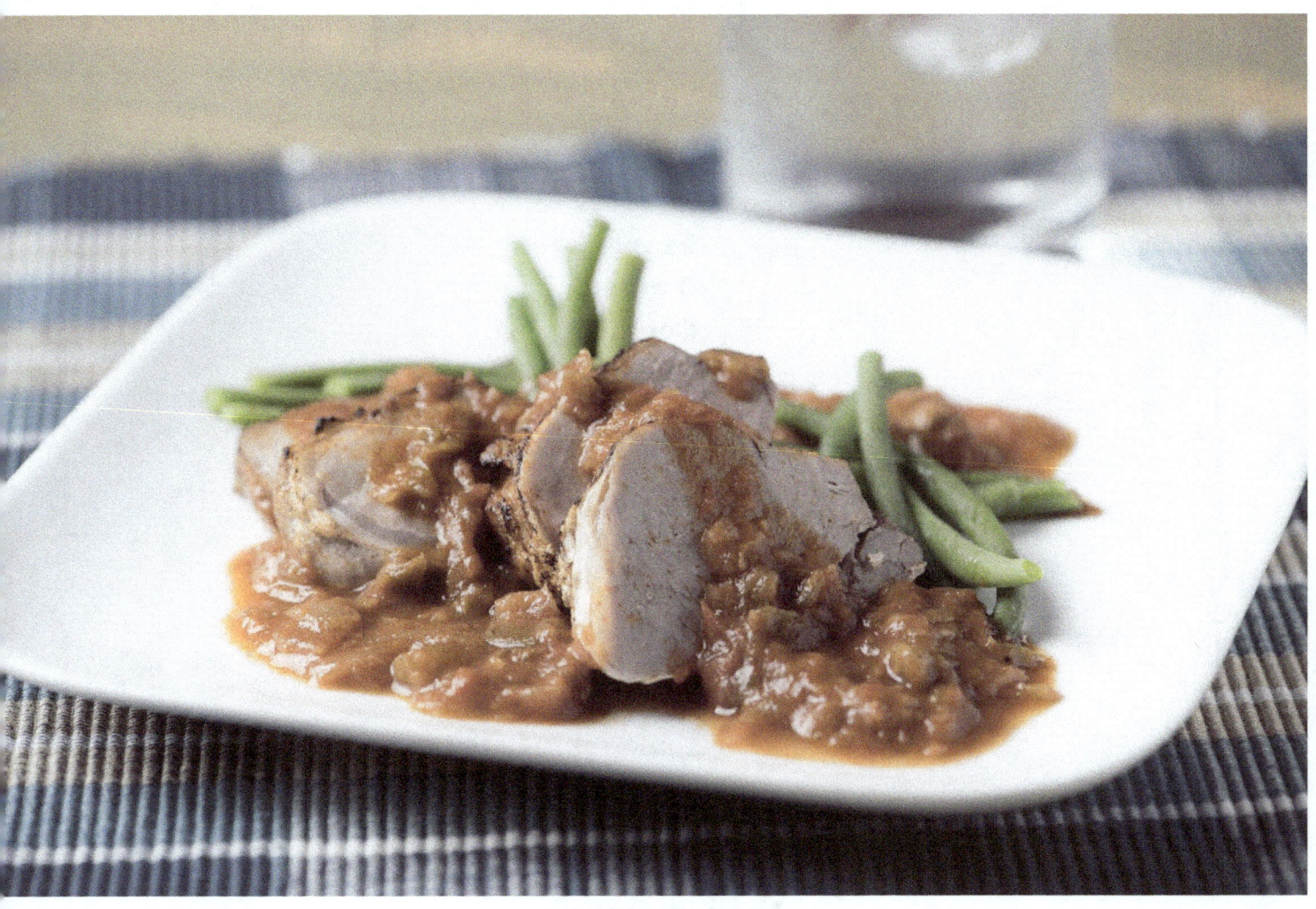

AMAZING RICE AND BEEF STUFFED TOMATOES

Prep:
20 mins
Cook:
35 mins
Total:
55 mins
Servings:
7
Yield:
7 stuffed tomatoes

INGREDIENTS:

7 tomatoes
1 cup water
1 cup instant rice
1 pound lean ground beef
1 yellow onion, chopped
1 clove garlic, diced
1 pinch garlic salt, or to taste
ground black pepper to taste
2 (15 ounce) cans tomato sauce
1 (6 fluid ounce) can tomato juice (Optional)

DIRECTIONS:

1

Preheat oven to 350 degrees F (175 degrees C).
Grease a 9x13-inch baking dish.

2

Cut tops from tomatoes and scoop out the pulp;
transfer pulp to a bowl and chop.
Reserve tops of tomatoes.

3

Bring water to a boil in a saucepan,
pour in the rice, and cover pan;
let stand until rice absorbs water, about 5 minutes.

4

Heat a large skillet over medium-high heat.
Cook and stir beef
in the hot skillet until browned
and crumbly, 5 to 7 minutes; drain and discard grease.
Mix cooked rice, onion,
garlic, garlic salt, and black pepper into ground beef;
add reserved tomato pulp and tomato sauce.
Bring the mixture to a boil, reduce heat to low, and simmer until
thickened, 10 minutes.

5
Set hollowed-out tomatoes into
the prepared baking
dish and fill each tomato with ground beef mixture.
If desired,
place tomato tops back on filled tomatoes.
Pour tomato juice over filled tomatoes
for extra juiciness.

6
Bake in the preheated oven until tomatoes
are tender and filling is hot, about 20 minutes.

NUTRITION FACTS:

249 calories; protein 16.9g; carbohydrates 27.8g; fat 8.6g;

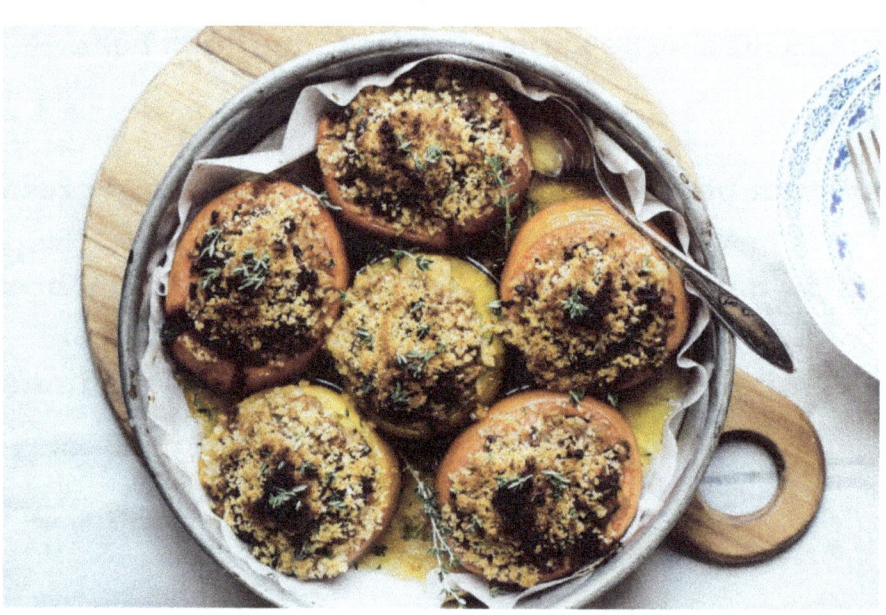

KOREAN BEEF WITH CAULI RICE

Prep:
10 mins
Cook:
10 mins
Total:
20 mins
Servings:
4
Yield:
4 servings

INGREDIENTS:

2 teaspoons sesame oil
1 pound lean ground beef
3 cloves garlic, minced
¼ cup soy sauce
1 tablespoon coconut sugar
¼ teaspoon ground ginger
¼ teaspoon ground black pepper
2 cups cauliflower rice
2 tablespoons chopped green onions
1 tablespoon sesame seeds

DIRECTIONS:

1

Heat sesame oil in a large skillet over medium-high heat. Cook and stir ground beef and garlic in the hot skillet until browned and crumbly, 5 to 7 minutes.

2

Combine soy sauce, coconut sugar, ginger, and black pepper in a bowl; whisk until well combined. Pour over ground beef; simmer until the sauce thickens, about 3 minutes.

3

Serve over cauliflower rice. Sprinkle with green onions and sesame seeds.

NUTRITION FACTS:

297 calories; protein 22.4g; carbohydrates 8.9g; fat 19.1g;

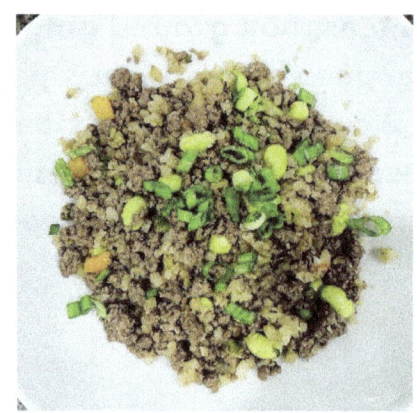

VEGGIE AND BEEF CHILI

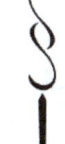

Prep:
25 mins
Cook:
45 mins
Total:
1 hr 10 mins
Servings:
8
Yield:
8 servings

INGREDIENTS:

1 pound lean ground beef
1 onion, chopped
1 green bell pepper, chopped
1 yellow bell pepper, chopped
1 carrot, diced
1 zucchini, diced
1 yellow squash, diced
1 (28 ounce) can crushed tomatoes
1 (16 ounce) can kidney beans, rinsed and drained
1 (16 ounce) can black beans, rinsed and drained
1 (15 ounce) can diced tomatoes
1 cup frozen white corn kernels

1 tablespoon minced garlic
1 ¼ tablespoons chili powder
1 tablespoon brown sugar
½ teaspoon paprika
½ teaspoon dried oregano
½ teaspoon ground cayenne pepper
½ teaspoon ground cumin
½ teaspoon salt
½ teaspoon ground black pepper

DIRECTIONS:

1
Break ground beef into small pieces
into a large pot over medium heat;
cook and stir until beginning to brown, 3 to 5 minutes.
Add onion, green bell pepper,
yellow bell pepper,
and carrot to ground beef;
cook and stir until the vegetables begin to soften,
5 to 7 minutes. Stir zucchini
and yellow squash into the beef mixture;
continue cooking until the beef is completely browned,
3 to 5 minutes more.
Drain excess liquid from
the pot and return to medium heat.

2
Stir crushed tomatoes, kidney beans,
black beans, diced tomatoes,
corn, and garlic into the beef mixture;
bring to a boil. Season mixture
with chili powder, brown sugar, paprika, oregano,
cayenne pepper, cumin, salt, and black pepper.

3
Reduce heat to low, place a cover on the pot,
and cook chili at a simmer for 30 minutes.

NUTRITION FACTS:

337 calories; protein 19.6g; carbohydrates 38.1g; fat 13g; cholesterol 42.6mg;

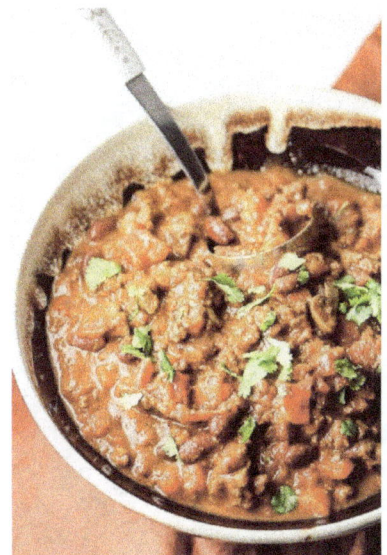

CHAPTER 7: VEGETABLE AND GRAIN RECIPES

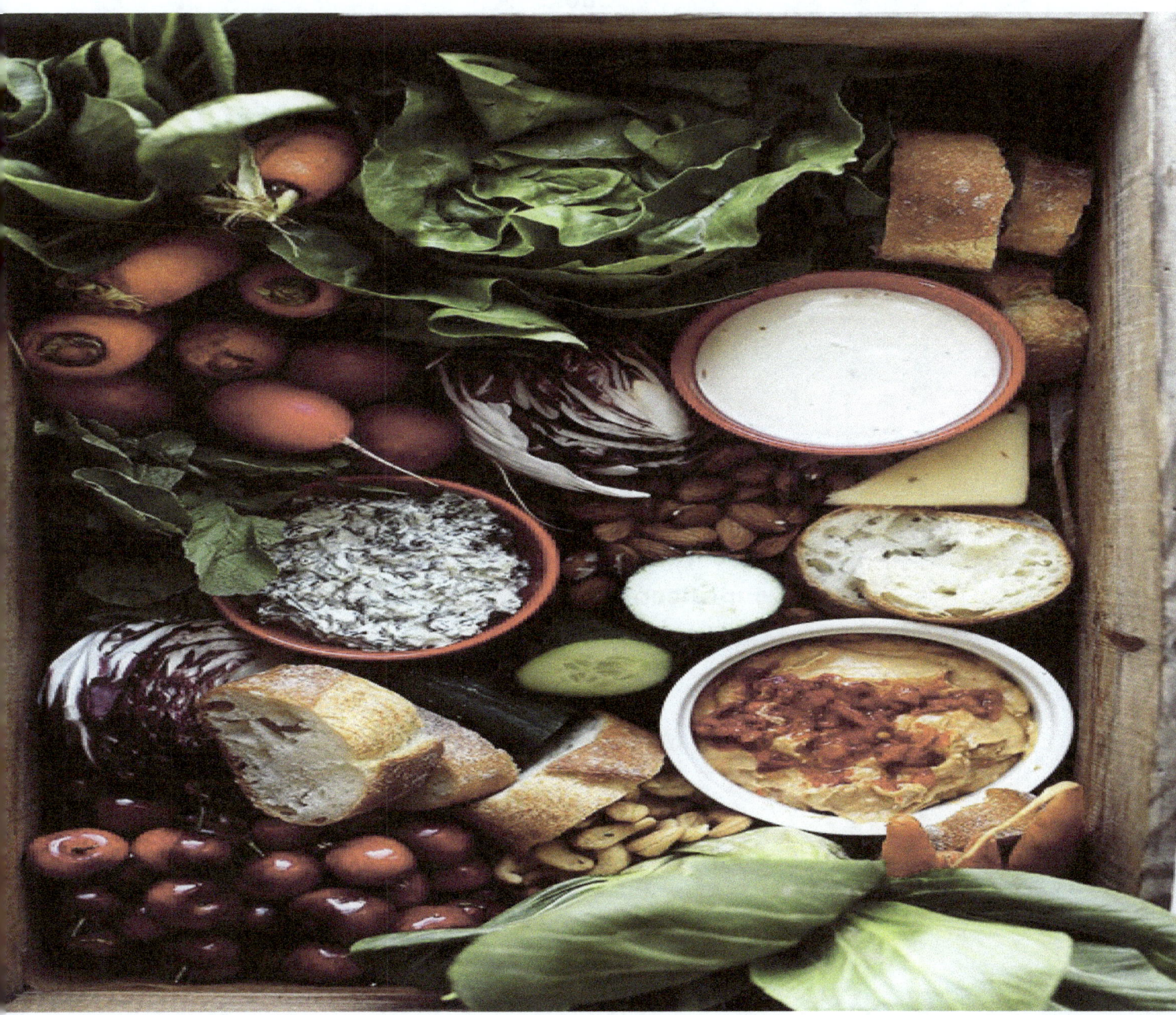

VEGGIE PITA PIZZA

Prep:
5 mins
Cook:
15 mins
Total:
20 mins
Servings:
1
Yield:
1 serving

INGREDIENTS:

1 pita bread round
1 teaspoon olive oil
3 tablespoons pizza sauce
½ cup shredded mozzarella cheese
¼ cup sliced crimini mushrooms
⅛ teaspoon garlic salt

DIRECTIONS:

1

Preheat grill for medium-high heat.

2

Spread one side of the pita with olive oil and pizza sauce.
Top with cheese and mushrooms,
and season with garlic salt.

3

Lightly oil grill grate.
Place pita pizza on grill, cover,
and cook until cheese completely melts,
about 5 minutes.

NUTRITION FACTS:

405 calories; protein 19.7g; carbohydrates 39.9g; fat 18g;

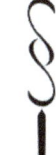

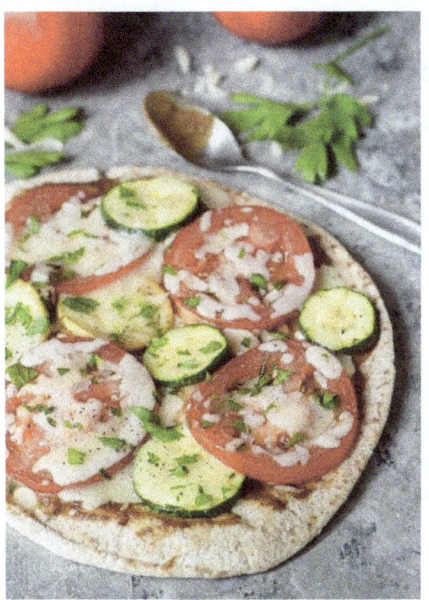

CURRY TOFU STIR-FRY

Prep:
10 mins
Cook:
25 mins
Total:
35 mins
Servings:
4
Yield:
4 main-dish servings

INGREDIENTS:

cooking spray
1 tablespoon chopped garlic
3 cups fresh spinach
2 tablespoons soy sauce
1 ½ tablespoons curry powder
1 teaspoon red pepper flakes (Optional)
1 pound extra-firm tofu, cut into 1-inch cubes
1 tablespoon vegetable oil
1 cup sliced fresh mushrooms

DIRECTIONS:

1

Preheat oven to 400 degrees F (200 degrees C).
Spray a baking sheet with baking spray;
arrange tofu in a single layer.

2

Bake tofu in preheated oven until evenly browned,
flipping after 10 minutes,
about 20 minutes total.

3

Heat vegetable oil in a wok or large skillet
over medium-high heat. Add mushrooms and garlic;
cook and stir until mushrooms are tender;
2 to 3 minutes. Add tofu, spinach, soy sauce,
and curry powder; cook and stir
until spinach is wilted; 3 to 5 minutes.
Sprinkle red pepper flakes over mixture.

NUTRITION FACTS:

143 calories; protein 11.4g; carbohydrates 6.6g; fat 9.4g;

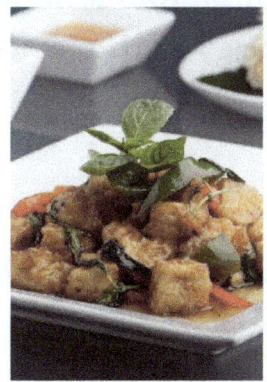

LENTILS AND SPINACH

Prep:
10 mins
Cook:
55 mins
Total:
1 hr 5 mins
Servings:
4
Yield:
4 servings

INGREDIENTS:

1 tablespoon vegetable oil
2 white onions, halved and sliced into 1/2 rings
3 cloves garlic, minced
½ cup lentils
2 cups water
1 (10 ounce) package frozen spinach
1 teaspoon salt
1 teaspoon ground cumin
freshly ground black pepper to taste
2 cloves garlic, crushed

DIRECTIONS:

1

Heat oil in a heavy pan over medium heat.
Saute onion for 10 minutes or so,
until it begins to turn golden.
Add minced garlic and
saute for another minute or so.

2

Add lentils and water to the saucepan.
Bring mixture to a boil. Cover, lower heat,
and simmer about 35 minutes,
until lentils are soft (this may take less time,
depending on your water and the lentils).

3

Meanwhile cook the spinach
in microwave according
to package directions.
Add spinach, salt and cumin
to the saucepan.
Cover and simmer until all is heated,
about ten minutes.
Grind in plenty of pepper
and press in extra garlic to taste.

NUTRITION FACTS:

165 calories; protein 9.7g; carbohydrates 24g; fat 4.3g;

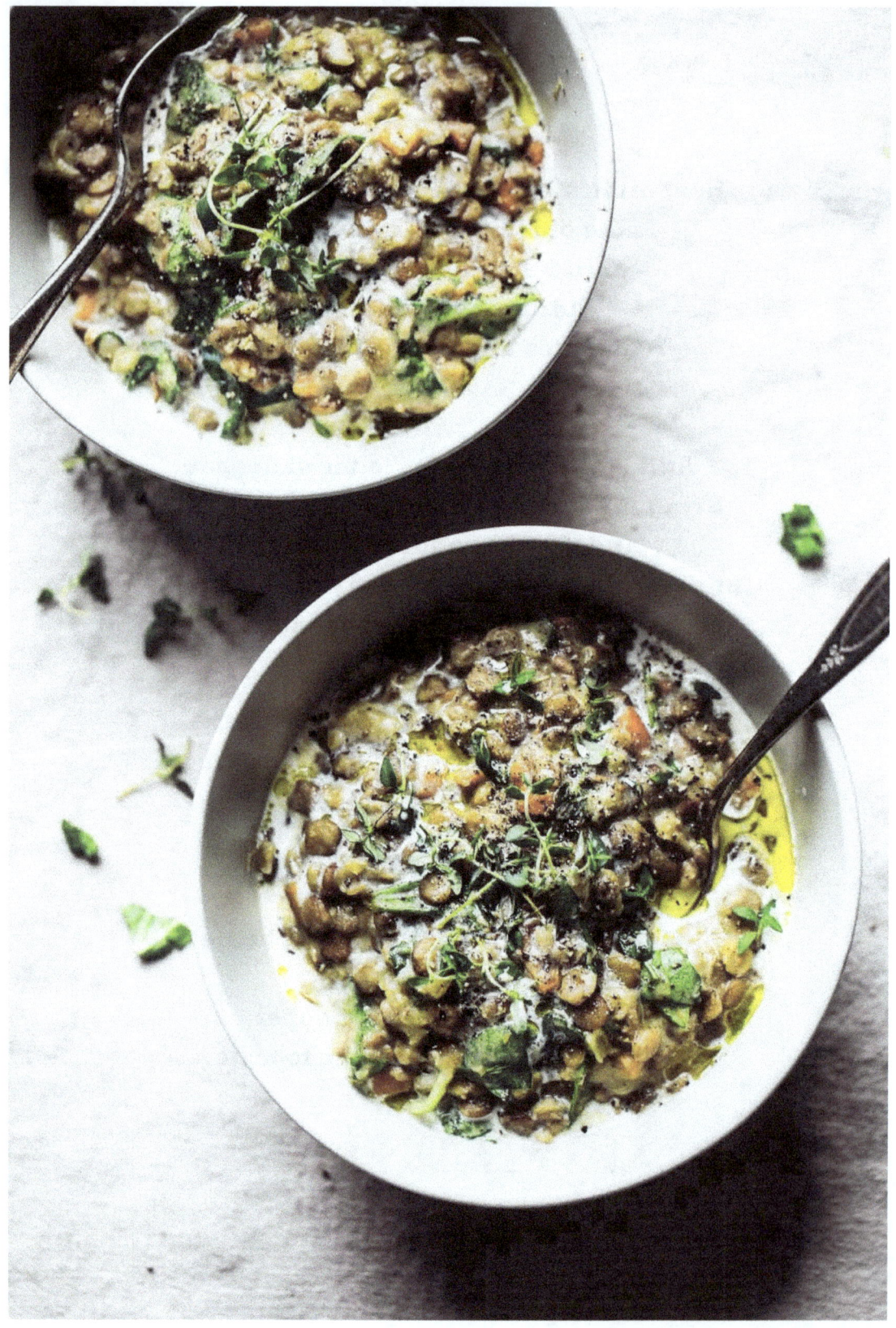

LIMA BEAN HUMMUS

Prep:
10 mins
Total:
10 mins
Servings:
6
Yield:
2 cups

INGREDIENTS:

3 tablespoons safflower oil, or more as needed
2 tablespoons tahini
2 tablespoons fresh lemon juice
1 tablespoon white vinegar
1 ½ teaspoons tamari (gluten-free soy sauce)
½ teaspoon ground cumin
½ teaspoon Celtic sea salt
½ teaspoon ground black pepper
1 clove garlic, minced
1 (1x4 inch) piece kombu seaweed (Optional)
1 pinch cayenne pepper
1 ¾ cups cooked lima beans
1 tablespoon chopped fresh parsley, or more to taste

DIRECTIONS:

1
Combine safflower oil, tahini, lemon juice,
vinegar, tamari, cumin, salt, black pepper,
garlic, kombu, and cayenne pepper
in a blender or food processor;
blend until smooth.
Add lima beans and blend until smooth,
adding more oil as desired.
Add parsley and pulse just until mixed.

NUTRITION FACTS:

204 calories; protein 6.8g; carbohydrates 23.3g; fat 9.7g;

VEGAN CHILI VERDE

Prep:
20 mins
Cook:
30 mins
Total:
50 mins
Servings:
6
Yield:
6 servings

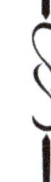

INGREDIENTS:

4 fresh tomatillos, husks removed and halved
4 cloves garlic
2 poblano peppers, tops, seeds, and membranes removed
3 tablespoons extra-virgin olive oil
1 medium white onion, diced
1 tablespoon dried oregano
1 tablespoon ground cumin
1 teaspoon chili powder
4 cups low-sodium vegetable broth, divided
1 (15 ounce) can low-sodium great Northern beans, rinsed and drained
1 (15 ounce) can low-sodium pinto beans, rinsed and drained
1 ½ cups chopped Tuscan kale
1 cup fresh corn kernels
¾ cup bulgur wheat
¾ teaspoon kosher salt

DIRECTIONS:

1
Set an oven rack 4 to 6 inches from
the heat source and preheat the oven's broiler.

2
Place tomatillos, garlic cloves,
and poblano peppers on a baking sheet.

3
Broil in the preheated oven until the peppers start
to blacken and blister, 6 to 8 minutes.
Remove garlic and transfer to a plate.
Turn tomatillos and peppers
over and broil until peppers are
blackened and tomatillos are soft, 5 to 6 minutes more.

4
Meanwhile, heat olive
oil in a large pot over medium heat until shimmering.
Add onion and cook, stirring frequently, until translucent,
about 5 minutes. Stir in oregano, cumin,
and chili powder; cook for 1 minute.
Add 3 cups vegetable broth,
great Northern beans,
pinto beans, kale, corn, bulgur wheat,
and salt. Return to a simmer.

5

Transfer roasted garlic, peppers, and tomatillos to a blender. Add remaining 1 cup vegetable broth. Cover and blend until just smooth. Pour into the simmering pot.

6

Simmer chili gently until bulgur is tender, 15 to 20 minutes.

NUTRTRITION FACTS:

315 calories; protein 12.6g; carbohydrates 49.7g; fat 8.9g; s

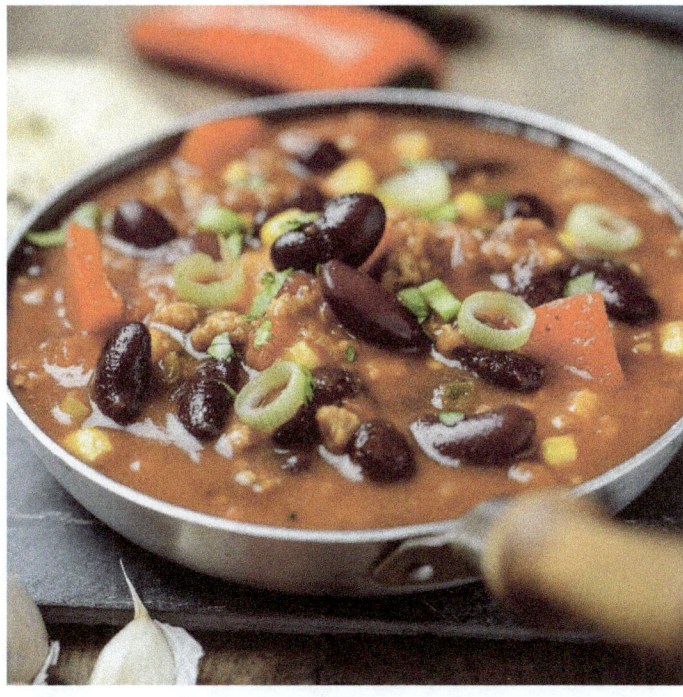

www.ingramcontent.com/pod-product-compliance
Lightning Source LLC
Chambersburg PA
CBHW081415080526
44589CB00016B/2544